CONDITIONING WITH IMAGERY FOR DANCERS

CONDITIONING WITH IMAGERY FOR DANCERS

DONNA KRASNOW AND JORDANA DEVEAU

THOMPSON EDUCATIONAL PUBLISHING, INC.
Toronto, Ontario

Information on how to obtain copies of this book is available at:
Website: http://www.thompsonbooks.com
E-mail: publisher@thompsonbooks.com
Telephone: (416) 766–2763
Fax: (416) 766–0398

Library and Archives Canada Cataloguing in Publication

Krasnow, Donna
Conditioning with imagery for dancers / Donna Krasnow, Jordana Deveau.

Includes bibliographical references and index.
ISBN 978-1-55077-207-4

1. Dancing injuries--Prevention. 2. Dance--Safety measures. 3. Imagery (Psychology). 4. Exercise. I. Deveau, Jordana, 1982- II. Title.

GV1782.3.K73 2010 792.802 C2010-906177-2

There is a C-I Training™ DVD series (beginning, intermediate, and advanced) and a teacher certification program. For information on ordering the DVD series or registering for the courses, visit www.citraining.com.

Production Editor: Katy Bartlett
Cover Design: Tibor Choleva
Copy Editor: Nina Paris
Proofreader: Caley Baker
Photography: Gary Ray Rush, www.garyrayrush.com
Cover Illustration: Martin Murphy, www.martinmurphy.ca

We acknowledge the support of the Government of Canada through the Book Publishing Industry Development Program for our publishing activities.

Printed in Canada. 1 2 3 4 5 6 14 13 12 11 10

TABLE OF CONTENTS

Part Two: Legwork and Core Support

Part Three: Flexibility Series

Part Four: Développé and Rond de Jambe Series

Part Five: Developing Turnout

Part Six: On Extension

Part Seven: Final Strength and Stretch

Section Three: Appendix

About the Authors

Donna Krasnow

Donna Krasnow is a professor in the Department of Dance at York University in Toronto, Canada, and has been an invited guest at many colleges, universities, and professional training institutions including Victorian College of the Arts in Melbourne, Australia, Arts Umbrella in Vancouver, and California State University, Northridge. She was the founding artistic director of Möbius Dance Company in San Francisco, California, and has performed and taught extensively in the United States, Canada, Australia, and Japan. Her primary artistic influence was Daniel Lewis, founding director of the Limón Institute in New York. In 1988, Donna became head of the modern division at the Canadian Children's Dance Theatre, under Artistic Director Deborah Lundmark, developing a curriculum for young dancers merging Limón-based modern dance with improvisation. Donna specializes in dance science research, concentrating on dance kinesiology, injury prevention, conditioning for dancers, motor learning and motor control, with a special emphasis on the young dancer. Her published articles can be found in many prestigious dance and performing arts journals. Donna conducts workshops and courses for dance teachers that focus on alignment and healthy dance training practices. She regularly presents her work at international conferences.

Jordana Deveau

Jordana Deveau is the associate artistic director of the Canadian Children's Dance Theatre, under Artistic Director Deborah Lundmark. Jordana is a dancer, educator, rehearsal director, and outreach workshop facilitator. In collaboration with Jesse Dell, she is co-artistic director of JD Dance, a contemporary dance company committed to creating and presenting socially-conscious work that communicates to a broad audience. She is a founding member of Event Horizon Dance, directed by Miranda Abbott. Jordana began her professional training with the Canadian Children's Dance Theatre in 1990, dancing in the company from 1994 to 2000. After leaving CCDT, she studied anthropology at the University of British Columbia. She has studied extensively with Donna Krasnow, and acted as her demonstrator and assistant in classes. As an independent artist she has performed in theatres and festivals in New York, Berlin, and across Canada.

Acknowledgements

Our thanks to the dancers in the photographs: Chad Clark, Jordana Deveau (courtesy of JD Dance), Kendra Epik, Ellis Martin-Wylie, Belinda McGuire (courtesy of José Limón Dance Company), Midori Mukai, Natasha Poon Woo, Meredith Thompson (courtesy of Danny Grossman Dance), and Samuel Xu.

Special thanks to Deborah Lundmark, artistic director of the Canadian Children's Dance Theatre, Daniel Lewis, Virginia Wilmerding, Samantha Lazzaro, and to our teachers and mentors throughout the years for their knowledge and support.

The conditioning work in C-I Training incorporates material and concepts from Fitt (1988); Friedman and Eisen (1980); Solomon (1988) and in classes with Ruth Solomon (1980–1982); and floor barre work by Zena Rommett, learned in classes with Ernest Pagano (1981–1983).

The sources for the imagery work include the following: Sweigard (1974); Bartenieff (1980); classes in Bartenieff Fundamentals with Sherri Barr (1993); Dowd (1990); and classes and private sessions with Irene Dowd (1991).

The exercises and imagery have been modified to enhance continuity throughout the process, and to emphasize the five principles of C-I Training, which will be described later. Additional source materials include postures and breath work from hatha yoga classes, Qi Gong, and exercises learned from physiotherapists during injury rehabilitation sessions.

Finally, students and colleagues over the years have made invaluable contributions to the ongoing evolution of C-I Training. This book would not be possible without the commitment and dedication of Jordana Deveau, collaborator in this manuscript.

This book is dedicated to our mothers, Harriet Krasnow-Katzen and Trixie Deveau, who always shine light on our paths, wherever the journey takes us.

There is a C-I Training™ DVD series (beginning, intermediate, and advanced) and a teacher certification program. For information on ordering the DVD series or registering for the courses, visit www.citraining.com.

Introduction

The importance of body conditioning for dance, athletics, and daily life is becoming increasingly recognized and valued by teachers, artistic directors, coaches, and medical practitioners. Dance educators and researchers are currently exploring what is essential for the dancer's training. Muscular strength and endurance, as well as flexibility can improve performance, reduce the risk of injuries, and enhance aesthetic beauty. It is becoming common for dancers to engage in methods—such as somatic practices and conditioning programs—outside of the traditional dance class setting to realize these goals.

For these changes in the body's physique to be beneficial, it is crucial that the brain learns how to "speak" to the muscles so that they are organized in more efficient ways. This is called neuromuscular patterning, or motor recruitment. When we dance or move about in daily life, it is rare that single muscles achieve a task; rather, it is the complex organization of multiple muscle groups that must be achieved. We refer to this as body integration, and it is the brain's job to establish patterns of muscle use involving core support, balanced muscle function, and the right amounts of muscle tension and release to optimize the movement without undue stress.

C-I Training™ (conditioning-with-imagery) is a body conditioning system designed specifically for dancers. It was developed with a focus on integrating the physical work in conditioning systems with the neuromuscular patterning intention of somatic practices. It incorporates exercises to develop muscular strength, endurance, and flexibility, as well as visualization and imagery work for movement re-education, alignment work, and mind-body integration and connectedness. C-I Training provides the dancer with an excellent method for warming up prior to class or rehearsal, as well as enhanced dance technique, and injury prevention through improved alignment and muscle balance.

Overview of Book Contents

The book is divided into seven parts:

- Fundamental Principles and Warm-Up
- Legwork and Core Support
- Flexibility Series
- Développé and Rond de Jambe Series
- Developing Turnout
- On Extension
- Final Strength and Stretch

Within each section, the reader will find descriptions of the exercises with accompanying imagery, the purpose of the exercise, applications and transfer to standing and travelling work, and additional notes for teachers. There is a developmental progression for the C-I Training system; however, the exercises can also be used individually within a dance class to enhance motor learning and skill acquisition. If done as a continuous progression, the transitions are specifically choreographed, with the goal of maintaining clear focus and concentration on the experience throughout the process.

How to Use this Book

The book is a valuable tool for both dancers and dance teachers, from recreational to elite levels of training. This system is excellent for a variety of age groups. With instruction and guidance from an experienced teacher, the early material can be taught to children as young as ten years old, or adults with little previous experience. A major advantage is that it provides a complete conditioning system that does not require equipment or a large space. For those who desire additional visual information, there are DVDs of the system at beginner, intermediate, and advanced levels, available at www.citraining.com.

If you are a dancer, start by reading the description of the exercise and studying the photographs provided with the text. You will find information on the physical form as well as the rhythmic structure of each one. Once the exercise is clear to you, begin to integrate the images that are described in the boxes in the margins. When learning C-I Training, begin with the first exercise in each section. As this exercise becomes familiar and easy for you, progress to more advanced variations. How fast you progress is entirely up to you and depends on previous training, how often you do the system, and your goals. To gain full benefit from this work, read the sections entitled "Purpose" and "Applications and Transfer to Standing and Travelling Work." When you return to your dance class, incorporate the images learned in specific C-I Training exercises when doing dance movements that are related.

If you are a teacher, the additional notes provided with each section highlight common difficulties that your students may encounter when first attempting the material, and describe modifications you may wish to include for individual student needs. There are examples of partner work and hands-on cueing, as well as explanations to enhance the transfer of the work to dance practice. There are also suggestions for ways to incorporate and refer to concepts learned in C-I Training when in dance class. These tools can be used when teaching new material to students, or when giving feedback to improve learned material.

Principles of Conditioning and Useful Terminology

There are several terms that are integral to the understanding of conditioning that will be simply and briefly described here. While these terms may not be specifically discussed in this text, the system was designed with these principles in mind. For more detailed explanations of this terminology, please refer to the excellent sources listed in the Bibliography starting on page 151.

- **Muscular strength** is the amount of tension that can be exerted by a muscle in a single maximum effort. Developing strength involves doing a relatively low number of repetitions of a task with a high level of effort.
- **Muscular endurance** is generally defined as the ability of a muscle to withstand fatigue during work at a specified intensity. In other words, it involves an extended duration—or a higher number of repetitions—of effort at a submaximal level. Note: Exercises that improve strength improve muscular endurance, but the reverse is not true.
- **Range of motion** refers to complete or full movement of a joint. For example, in a joint such as the elbow, the range of motion would be the distance between the fully flexed position and the extended position. Structures influencing range of motion include muscles, tendons, ligaments, skeletal (joint) structure, and other connective tissues. There are also neurological factors (such as heightened emotional states) that can influence range of motion. The term "hypermobility" is used to refer to bodies that have extreme ligamentous laxity, and can move joints beyond what is considered normal range.
- **Flexibility** refers to the suppleness or available length of a muscle to provide good range of motion. Dancers are expected to have significantly more flexibility than the general population.
- **Frequency** refers to how often one performs an exercise session.
- **Duration** refers to the length of time that an exercise session lasts.
- **Intensity** refers to the degree of effort exerted during an exercise session.
- **Periodization** refers to the process of structuring training into phases over time.
- **Specificity** refers to making the exercises relevant and appropriate to the activity for which the individual is practising.
- The **Overload Principle** states that to improve conditioning, the exercises must exceed levels of previous capacity. This increase in loading must be progressive, that is, gradually enhanced with each session. Abrupt changes can lead to injury and burnout.
- **Proprioception** refers to the sense of knowing where the body is in space; it is both a conscious and a nonconscious perception of motion and spatial orientation. It not only includes stationary

positioning of body parts, but also the speed and direction of movement. This information is sent to the brain from neurons (nerve cells) in muscles, tendons, ligaments, joints, and (some scientists believe) messages from the skin. Dancers call this their "kinesthetic sense" or "kinesthetic awareness." Balancing mechanisms and the ability to remain centred under bright stage lights depend on good proprioception.

- In this text, **neural recruitment** refers to the activation of muscle fibres by neurons located in the central nervous system (CNS) (brain and spinal cord), and the peripheral nervous system (the nerve pathways that lead from the CNS to the rest of the body). Muscles are entirely dependent on nerve impulses to contract, though this may come from voluntary or nonconscious brain signals.
- **Neural release** refers to the decreased activation of muscles, at times leading to full relaxation of muscles, when the neural impulses diminish or cease.

The terms **tonic** (slow twitch) and **phasic** (fast twitch) are used to describe muscle fibres and the nerve cells that fire on these fibres. Muscles that are primarily tonic have slowly contracting fibres that are adapted for low intensity, ongoing activation. Muscles that are primarily phasic have rapidly contracting fibres adapted for high-intensity, intermittent activation. In general, the muscles that are designed to support our posture in sitting, stance, and locomotion all day are tonic or slow twitch muscles. Examples are the neck muscles holding up the head, and the lumbar extensors supporting the spine. These muscles tend to be closer to the skeleton, and do not require conscious thought or voluntary contraction to achieve the task. Muscles that are more superficial on the body tend to be phasic or fast twitch, and do require conscious decisions to activate. These muscles are movers, not postural supports, and work in short bursts. When teachers ask students to engage specific muscles to correct alignment, it is common that the students will activate superficial muscles, as these are more easily recruited through conscious effort. However, this is only a quick fix, and does not teach the brain how to activate the appropriate deeper muscles that need to be working for correct alignment.

The **sympathetic** and **parasympathetic** nervous systems together make up the autonomic system, and regulate the ongoing function of heart rate, digestion, respiration rate, salivation, perspiration, and levels of arousal. When the body and its systems are highly aroused, the sympathetic nervous system is called into action, which is often referred to as "fight or flight." When the system is calmed, the parasympathetic nervous system responds, which is referred to as "rest and repose" or "rest and digest." The somatic practices (to be described later) rely on bringing the mind to a state of awareness and calm in order to engage the parasympathetic system, thereby facilitating a state of relaxation. In this state, it is possible to achieve subtle neuromuscular changes without the interference of large, power muscles.

Principles of C-I Training

The following five principles, developed from the above conditioning ideas and from somatic concepts, were incorporated into the C-I Training design. These five principles emphasize the merger of physical conditioning and neuro-muscular repatterning that is at the heart of C-I Training.

- **Integration Principle**: The whole body is integrated into each activity, even the most minimal movement. While the body might be relaxed in a given minimal movement, awareness of the interconnectedness of all the body segments is crucial. This principle includes the idea of mind-body integration, and suggests that the mind is focused on how the task is being performed, not just on the form or sequencing of the exercise.
- **Increasing Principle**: Low levels of contractile activity develop to higher levels of muscular work, and small range of motion develops to greater range of motion. This principle applies to the progression of the system over time, as well as within a given session. Additionally, there is development during the sessions from simple tasks to compound and complex activities.
- **Alternating Principle**: The sequence of exercises alternates work in muscular strength, muscular endurance, and flexibility. It alternates work in antagonist muscle groups (muscles performing opposite actions at a given joint), upper/lower body work, and left/right body work. This principle reinforces the concept of balanced muscle function, ensuring that attention is given to each area of conditioning, and to antagonist muscle groups to promote balanced and efficient function.
- **Specificity Principle**: The program incorporates tasks that relate as closely as possible to dance practice. This principle is based on the hypothesis that muscle patterns and balanced muscle function learned in a dance-specific context will more likely relate to muscle use required in dance performance, and also the notion that imagery that is dance-related will be more applicable with exercises that are also dance-related.
- **Attentiveness Principle**: Attention is directed to those aspects of an exercise that affect the quality of work, such as movement process, breath, timing, and transitions. This principle is derived from the goal of wanting to affect the qualitative and experiential aspects of dance and everyday movement, as well as modify the musculoskeletal structure for improved efficiency and injury prevention.

Additional Elements

Musicality, in terms of phrasing and rhythm, is incorporated throughout the system. This was intended as one approach to satisfying the specificity principle. Variations in tempo and rest times are encouraged.

Experiential Anatomy, the process of learning about the anatomical functioning of the body through experience and sensation, is paramount in this work. Students will receive greater benefit from C-I Training if they are provided with an understanding of how and why the exercises and images function, rather than simply learning the form. This process leads to a journey of self-discovery and knowledge about movement and function that will inform students' dance practice.

Imagery

The use of imagery is a psychological activity that evokes the physical characteristics of an object or dynamic event absent from one's immediate experience. Imagery does not necessarily involve visualizing a particular movement sequence. There are several categories of images, not all mutually exclusive: visual and kinesthetic, direct and indirect, internal and external, metaphorical and anatomical. Images can be directional, such as the lines-of-movement imagery in Ideokinesis, or global, which involve totality, creating an overall state, such as "imagine that the body is floating in water."

Some of the early somatic pioneers, such as Irmgard Bartenieff, Lulu Sweigard, and Mabel Todd, relied on imagery as an important part of the process of changing alignment and movement patterns. They discussed the importance of balanced muscle function for improved alignment, and subsequently better biomechanical efficiency, fewer injuries, and greater range of motion. They claimed that changes to the balance of antagonist muscles must happen on the neurological level, not the muscle-tissue level. It is imagery operating nonconsciously that creates the neuromuscular responses necessary to alter alignment and to carry out movement in efficient ways. The idea of forming mental concepts to facilitate muscle function rather than voluntarily contracting the muscles, has formed the basis of some current work in dance training, particularly in the area of alignment and movement patterning.

The use of imagery during specific conditioning exercises is less common than its use in somatic practices or in dance classes and rehearsals. It might seem that conditioning is, by its nature, mechanistic and therefore inaccessible to imagery; however, imagery can provide an ideal method for neuromuscular re-patterning while strength and flexibility are being enhanced. Many teachers have witnessed the dance student who does hours of abdominal strength work, hip flexor stretching, and lumbar extensor stretching, and yet comes to dance class still exhibiting lordotic (swayback) posture. Imagery can offer a method, during the conditioning exercises, to inform these muscle groups at the nonconscious level about how they work as an integrated whole to align the pelvis in relation to the spine and legs.

Balanced Muscle Function

C-I Training has been designed to merge conditioning and imagery to address the three components of balanced muscle function: strength and flexibility of a given muscle, balanced use of antagonist muscles, and efficient motor recruitment. The first component is strength and flexibility within a given muscle or muscle group. There are exercises in the system to develop increased strength in the hamstrings, which tend to be far more flexible than strong. Similarly, there are exercises to increase flexibility of the hip flexor muscles, a muscle group that can often be strong but tight. These exercises attempt to create a balance in the relative strength and flexibility within each of the muscle groups.

The second component concerns balanced or efficient function of antagonist muscles around joints. For example, C-I Training includes various exercises to increase abdominal strength and to enhance flexibility and release in the lumbar spinal extensors and in the hip flexors. Imagery work is included to facilitate correct alignment of the pelvis, and to encourage this alignment without excessive and unnecessary tension in the gluteals and quadriceps.

The third component of balanced muscle function is efficient motor recruitment. There are several exercises that involve extending the hip and knee joints while plantar flexing the ankles (i.e., straightening the legs and pointing the feet). The imagery used in these instances involves reaching the feet out in the space (directed spatial intention), while visualizing the inner thighs gathering or being drawn together as two magnets, thereby encouraging hip adductor use and inhibiting quadriceps overuse. A second example involves a hip flexion series that works on both hip flexor strength and use of the outward rotators. The imagery includes visualizing the sacrum weighted and heavy on the floor as the flexion occurs, and then visualizing the spine elongating along the floor as the abdominals hollow during the return of the limb to extension. The imagery is designed to encourage appropriate pelvic stabilization as a component of core support for standing hip flexion movements, such as grand battement devant.

Transfer of Training

Many dance educators are aware of the problem of transfer of training, that is, the transfer of material from exercises to dance practice, and transfer from one setting or context to another. For example, it is a common belief that enhanced strength or flexibility in a conditioning program will transfer to improved skills, such as jumping or leg extensions. It is also sometimes assumed that realignment work done in body therapy or physiotherapy sessions will have significant impact on the dancer's alignment habits when he or she returns to class or rehearsal. However, many educators have witnessed the transfer problems that dancers encounter. The dancers will improve in strength or flexibility levels, or exhibit noted changes in alignment during a body therapy session, but show little change in either skills or alignment habits during dance classes or rehearsals. If dancers are to be encouraged to do increased training outside of dance classes and rehearsals, whether weight training, yoga, or body therapy work, how can educators and researchers ensure that the results of these practices can be accessed during complex dancing? The philosophy of C-I Training proposes that combining conditioning work with specific images that can be used during complex dance movements might assist in the transfer process.

The imagery used in C-I Training can be directly applied to actual dance practice. For example, images are introduced while performing développés and rond de jambes while lying on the floor that encourage core support for the leg gestures. The use of the floor along with the imagery encourages lumbo-pelvic stability during full range of motion at the hip. In using these same images during stance, the dancer can re-experience that central stability to support the gesture. The conditioning work has provided the appropriate strength and range of motion to achieve this task. Another important aspect of C-I Training is that it focuses on whole body connections, not isolating one muscle group from the rest of the system. This full integration allows for transferability to a standing and/or travelling context.

The following is another example demonstrating how the C-I Training system uses imagery to affect neuromuscular patterning during conditioning exercises. One of the concerns in teaching abdominal strength work is to assist the dancer in engaging the deeper abdominals, including the internal and external obliques and the transverse abdominals, for better core support during dancing. While doing pelvic tilts, as well as a variety of other strength exercises for abdominals, the dancer visualizes a row of elastics or rubber bands that attach to the pubic bone at their lower ends. The upper ends are gathered to a point so that the elastics form a triangle. This upper point is then attached to the lower back directly behind the navel. As the dancer exhales, the elastics shorten, drawing the pubic bone towards the low back, or "hollowing" the anterior pelvis. This image can be extended to work on proper execution of eccentric abdominal use. The dancer can move from the pelvic tilt to an overcurve, or hyperextension of the spine. Rather than simply relaxing the abdominals, the elastics can be visualized as remaining taut and elongating, thus giving resistance through eccentric abdominal work to the contraction of the spine extensors. This co-contraction is important for protection of the low back in movements such as arabesque, and grand jeté in which the back leg is required to lift during the landing. Finally, this same image can be applied to core support during stance when no pelvic movement is desired. By visualizing this row of elastics maintaining a connection between the pubic bone and the lumbar spine, the dancer can effectively stabilize the pelvis during dance movements such as pliés, relevés, and leg gestures.

Conclusion

It is now understood that the most efficient systems for enhancing dance technique and preventing injury address both the re-patterning work done in the somatic context, and the muscular-skeletal alterations achieved in conditioning work. These systems approach the study of motor control by suggesting that it is imperative to consider both the mechanical and the neurological perspectives in altering or training balance, locomotion, and a variety of dance skills. Further, it is the interaction of these systems that determines the efficacy of resulting motor patterns. It is this goal of addressing multiple systems that propelled the development of C-I Training as an alternative training system for dancers.

PART ONE FUNDAMENTAL PRINCIPLES AND WARM-UP

1

Opening Remarks

This section introduces the fundamental principles that support all of C-I Training. One of the primary components of this type of work is that dancers and dance students will be receiving information aurally, and sensing kinesthetically, rather than having most of the information provided visually. This can be a difficult adjustment in the beginning, particularly for very young students. After the Neutral Pelvis Lesson, it begins with the body's periphery, and then moves to the core. The reason for this choice is that working with the feet and arms is both tactile and visible. At the beginning of a movement session, especially for younger students, starting with core work immediately can be too subtle and too deep in the body for an easily accessible kinesthetic experience. Core work requires a depth of concentration that rarely occurs at the start of class. The use of breath underlies the entire system. First, on a physical level, breathing affects muscle function and can assist in releasing excess tension, and second, on a mental level, it brings the attention to the inner landscape.

A – Neutral Pelvis Lesson

Purpose

The primary purpose of the Neutral Pelvis Lesson is to establish the organization of the pelvis and lumbar spine that will be used throughout the C-I Training. This sequence is not intended to strengthen or stretch particular muscle groups; rather, it is an awareness exercise, designed to encourage recruitment of deep muscles that will support this dynamic alignment. When the dancer is working in neutral pelvis, these muscles are working with maximum efficiency. In a general sense, learning to work in neutral pelvis has advantages for injury prevention. The anterior pelvic tilt (swayback) causes chronic stress to the lumbar spine, while posterior pelvic tilt (tucking under) can create strain and long-term problems for the psoas. Any chronic misalignment in the pelvis can have repercussions for the knees and lower legs.

The series of exercises in the Neutral Pelvis Lesson also functions as a gentle warm-up without weight bearing for the lumbar spine and the hip joints. The goal of doing *Side-to-Side Rolling* and *Open and Close the Book* with as little effort as possible is to create space in the joints of the spine, particularly the articular facet joints.

It can be difficult for movement concepts practised at a slow, sustained dynamic to transfer to faster movement using momentum. Adding variations to the neutral pelvis exercises, such as altering tempo and exploring various dynamics, can assist this process.

1) Finding Neutral Pelvis

Start by lying on the back (supine) with the arms and legs extended, arms at the sides of the body. Focus on allowing the breath to be natural and the body segments to lie easefully with as little tension as possible. While inhaling, imagine the breath filling the body, and sense how it releases tension in the muscles on the exhale. Image the pubic bone directly above the tailbone (coccyx), and the back of the head, rib cage, and sacrum heavy and in contact with the floor. There will be spaces under the neck (cervical spine) and low back (lumbar spine), due to the natural curves of the spine. This organization of the pelvis is neutral pelvis in the supine position.

IMAGERY

Throughout the Neutral Pelvis Lesson, the image of the weighted sacrum and tailbone dropping to the floor can help to maintain the natural lumbar curve. For those dancers who see the body spatially, the image of the pubic bone resting directly above the tailbone can be useful. Expanding this image to include the sitz bones (ischial tuberosities), if there were a light shining out the bottom of this diamond (pubic bone, tailbone, and sitz bones), the light would shine directly onto the feet, not up towards the ceiling, or down towards the floor.

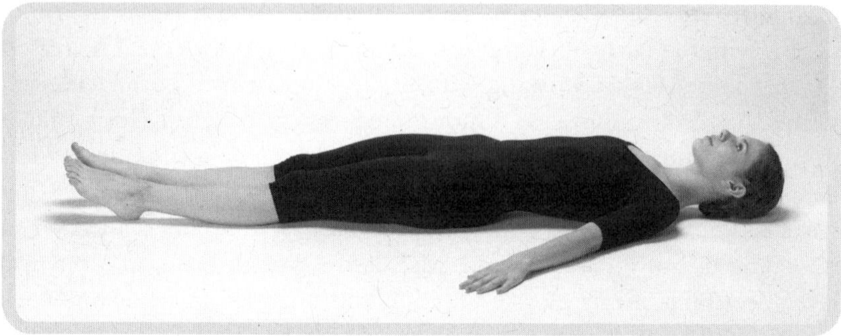

2) Parallel Legs Sliding

Place the hands on the floor or at the waist so that the palms rest on the iliac crests of the pelvis. Draw the thighs towards the pelvis by bending the knees, allowing the feet to stand in parallel on the floor (neutral stance). Be conscious of maintaining the organization of the pelvis during this action; if the pelvis tilts anteriorly (increased lumbar space) or tucks (decreased lumbar space), repeat the reach and draw of the legs several times, until the action can be done while keeping the pelvis quiet. The hands on the waist can provide external feedback as to how quiet the pelvis remains during this action of the legs, and should be used as light touch, not to hold the pelvis still.

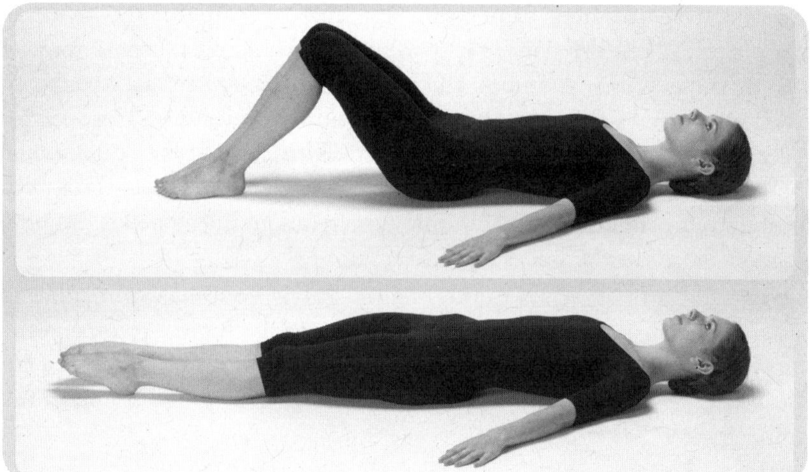

3) Side-to-Side Rolling

Move the arms so that they rest on the floor at shoulder height. Roll both legs to one side, lowering them to the floor easily, allowing the pelvis to rotate in that direction to accommodate full range. Then roll the legs back to the parallel stance position, imagining weight in the sacrum, and experiencing the space under the lumbar spine. Roll the legs to the other side, and back to centre again. This action can be done several times, always establishing neutral pelvis in the stance position, not rounding the lumbar spine so that it drops to the floor (posterior pelvic tilt).

IMAGERY

As the legs roll from side to side, one can image a magnet on the sacrum that is drawn to the floor during the return to neutral stance.

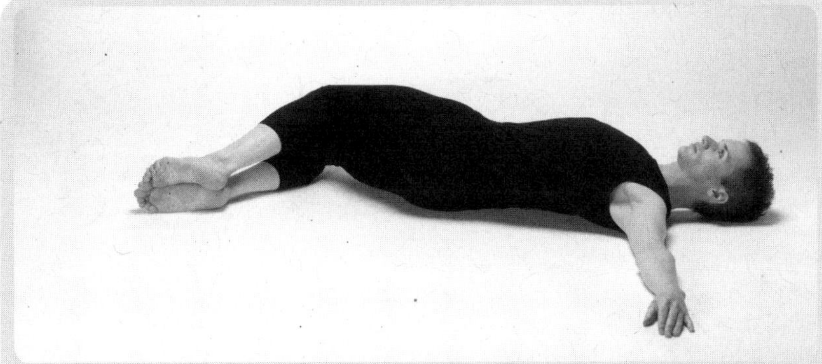

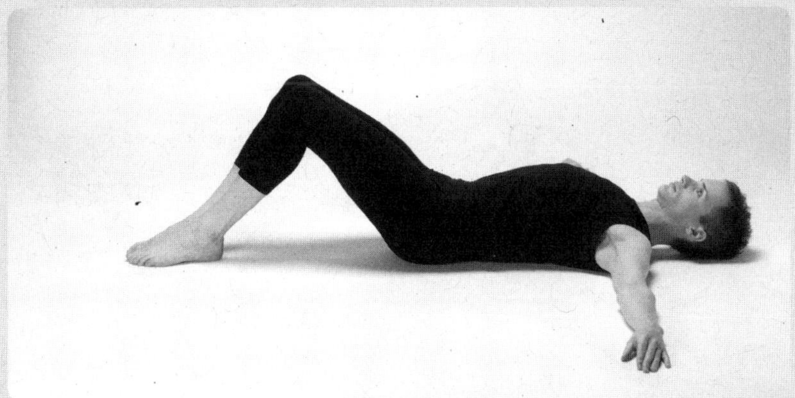

4) Open and Close the Book

The same action can be done with a slight variation. Start with both legs to one side. Move the top leg to the opposite side like a book (or a clam) opening, and when it has gone to its full range, bring the other leg across to meet it, like the book (or clam) closing. Go side to side with this action of one leg initiating, the second leg following. Observe that the legs will be in the fully open diamond position when the pelvis is centred. Once again, using the image of weighted sacrum, establish a neutral pelvis. Finish the process back in neutral parallel stance, knees to the ceiling, feet on the floor.

IMAGERY

In all of the exercises in which the legs slide out along the floor (#2, #5, and #6), imagine the front of the hip joints made of taffy, which softens and elongates as the leg lengthens.

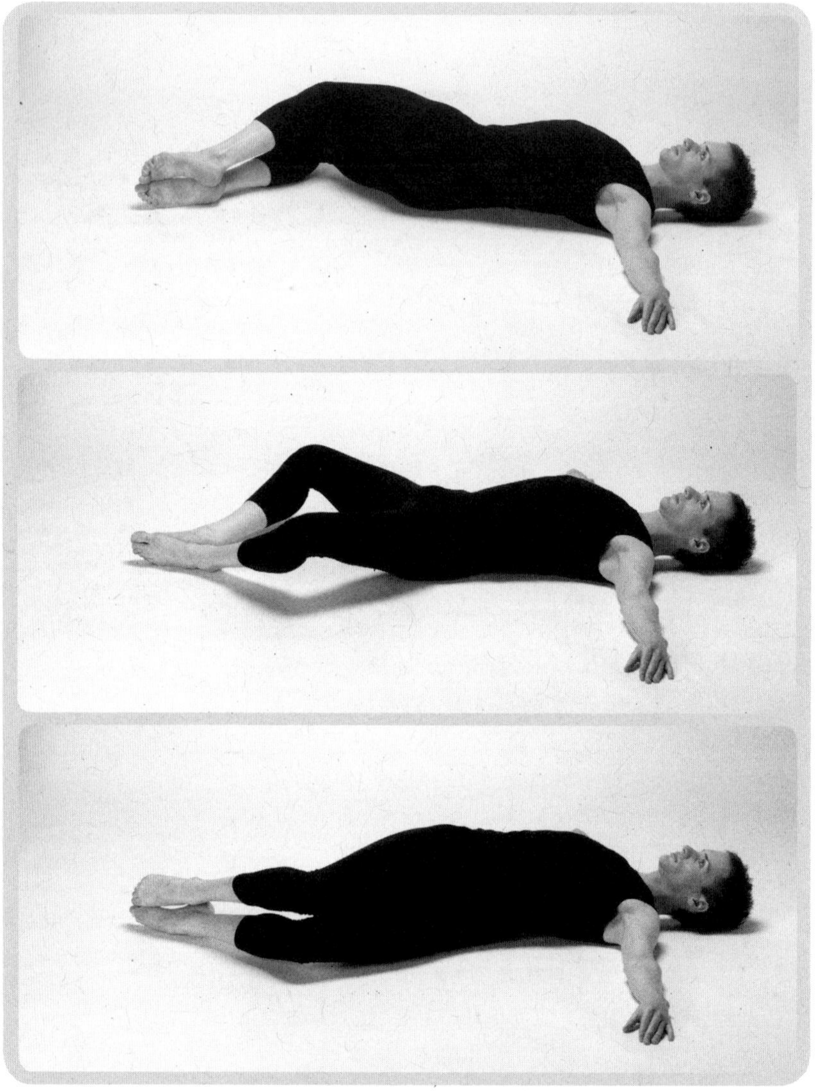

5) Turned Out Legs Sliding

Step #2 can now be repeated from the open diamond, hands at the waist, and heels staying in contact with the floor, with feet relaxed, so neutral pelvis can be established with hip and knee flexion and extension, but now in external rotation of the hips. As before, repeat the sliding of the legs in and out as many times as needed until the pelvis remains quiet, and the action is easeful.

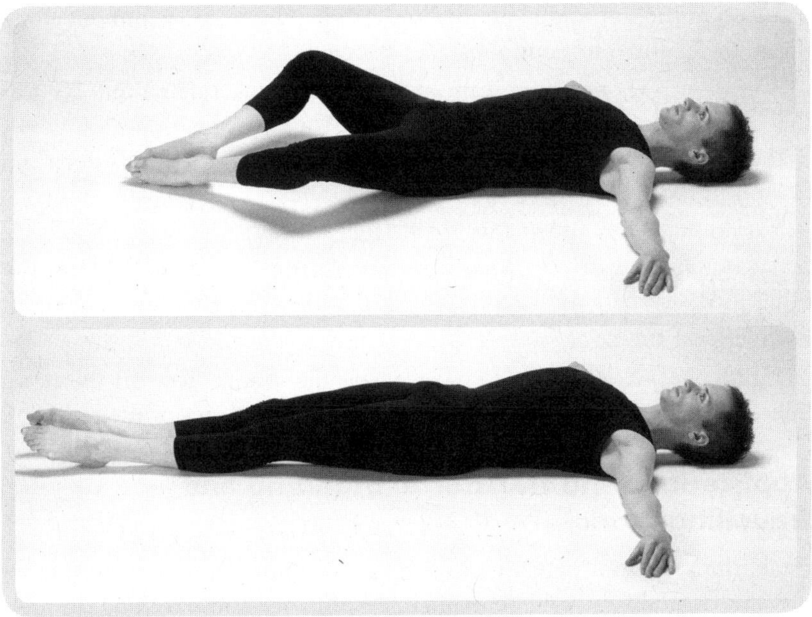

IMAGERY

For *Turned Out Legs Sliding*, imagine that the heels are glued together, and the gluteus maximus (buttocks) muscles soften and elongate down the backs of the legs as the legs slide out, in order to avoid tightening these muscles. Imagine the buttocks like unbaked bread dough that spreads into the floor as the legs slide out.

6) Walking in Space – Hip Flexion

From neutral stance, bring one thigh towards the chest, foot releasing off the floor, remaining parallel. The knee can be completely relaxed so that the joint is folded comfortably. The image of a weighted sacrum dropping more deeply into the floor as the hip flexes can assist in maintaining the neutral pelvis, rather than tucking under, which is a common tendency in hip flexion. Return this foot to the floor, conscious of the organization of the spine and pelvis, and repeat on the other side. Do several alternating repetitions, until hip flexion can be accomplished easily with a neutral pelvis.

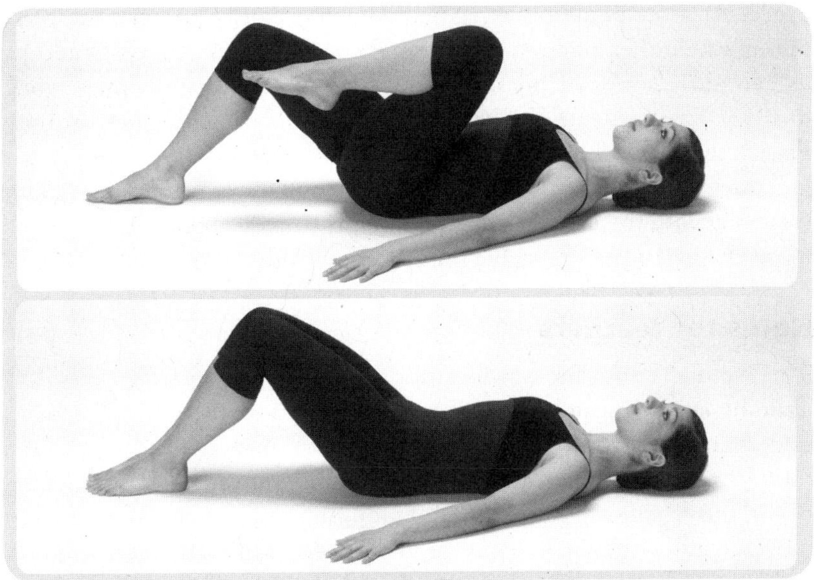

IMAGERY

With the hip flexion in parallel or *Walking in Space*, imagine a fishing line with the reel at the inside crease of the hip socket near the pubic bone, and the end of the line attached to the inside of the knee joint. Then reel it in to flex the hip.

Note: This image is intended to encourage hip flexion through use of the psoas, rather than the rectus femoris and/or tensor fasciae latae, which can cause the femur to drift laterally, and create excess tension in standing leg work. Using an image derived from spatial intention, see the knee moving in the direction of the outer sternum, not towards the shoulder joint.

Variation 1 - Increased range of motion for the hamstrings: Instead of a soft, folded knee, repeat the hip flexion series with a long, parallel attitude.

Variation 2 - Altering the tempo and dynamics: Starting from neutral stance, on a quick four-count rhythm, slide one leg along the floor 1;

bring up to the soft folded hip flexion 2; slide it back down and out along the floor 3; return to neutral parallel stance 4.

Variation 3 (For more advanced dancers only) - Turned out: Repeat the same series as Variation 2, but start in the open diamond; on count 2, the folded leg aims towards the shoulder, so that there is a deep hip flexion in hip abduction.

Variation 4 (For more advanced dancers only) - Repeat *Walking in Space*, but instead of returning one foot to the floor before lifting the other foot, alternate the feet in time, so that there are phases of time with both legs off the floor.

Finish the Neutral Pelvis Lesson in parallel stance, feet on the floor, knees towards the ceiling, arms resting easily at the sides of the body.

Applications and Transfer to Standing and Travelling Work

Establishing neutral pelvis lying supine does not necessarily guarantee that this organization will be maintained in stance and travelling through space. However, the experience and awareness gained through this lesson can facilitate the process. In stance, locate the pubic bone and the tailbone through tactile sensation. Play with moving the pelvis so that the pubic bone alternates between being higher than the tailbone, and then lower than the tailbone. Eventually arrive at the point where the two bones are level in relation to the floor. (Note: This is the same relationship as lying on the floor and having the pubic bone directly above the tailbone.) Maintain an awareness of the breathing throughout this exploration. Some dancers may respond to additional feedback, such as visual reinforcement using the mirror, or aural feedback from a teacher or another dancer. At some point, however, neutral pelvis should be achieved solely through kinesthetic awareness. The next stage of this process would be to execute a series of pliés, relevés, tendus, and other standing work, focusing on the neutral pelvis, and using the various images to assist. Finally, the work should progress to travelling material, reinforcing the kinesthetic experience of the neutral pelvis, and the assisting images. Play creatively with the images so that they apply to movements that are faster, more challenging, and involve shift of weight through space.

Notes for Teachers

The Neutral Pelvis Lesson does not need to be done with every C-I Training lesson. It can be done for the first few lessons, until the dancers understand how to do the C-I Training work in neutral pelvis. If, at a future time, the dancers are no longer consistently maintaining neutral pelvis, this lesson can be repeated. Through both somatic sensation and movement, this lesson is a way to get a sense of what neutral pelvis is, and how to move while maintaining it with minimal tension. In some cases, excessive tightness or tension in the back of the neck will cause a backward tilt of the head, lifting the chin in the lying supine position. In these cases, it is recommended that a flat pillow be used under the head until this area can be stretched over time.

B – Additional Preparations

Purpose

In dance, we learn to articulate our legs distinctly from movements of the pelvis and to articulate our arms distinctly from movements of the upper spine and scapulae. Seemingly paradoxical, dance requires the arms and legs to be connected to the spine and pelvis, but at the same time, we want to be able to move the limbs independently, with the appearance of isolation. There is tremendous unseen stabilization work going on internally to accomplish this way of working. These preparatory lessons are designed to introduce these concepts.

The Big X introduces the idea of the connection of the limbs to the core of the body. It also begins to open up the front of the hips for easeful neutral pelvis work. If the hip flexors are holding excess tension, the pelvis cannot align correctly, and will be forced into anterior tilt. Often, dancers will use unnecessary gripping in the gluteus maximus to address this misalignment. This is inefficient. *Rocking the Boat* establishes the release of tension in the neck and upper back. *Angels in the Snow* focuses on freeing upper limb movement and maintaining ease through the neck and shoulders.

1) The Big X – Core Initiation

Extend the arms and legs out along the floor, so that the body forms a large X. Imagine a magnet under the navel, drawing it towards the floor. While exhaling, fold to one side of the body, drawing the elbows and knees together into full spinal flexion, allowing the arms and legs to stay as much as possible in contact with the floor. While inhaling, gently open back out into the X, like the spokes of a wheel expanding. Repeat several times, alternating sides. A second variation does the same folding action, but the extension into the X is initiated by reaching the top leg out along the back low diagonal on the floor, until this reaching action pulls the body onto the back. Repeat, alternating sides several times, and finish in parallel stance.

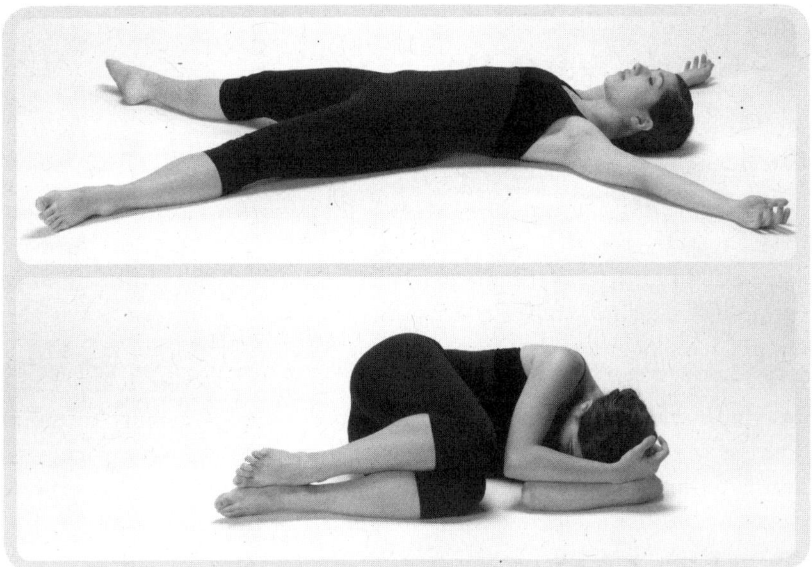

IMAGERY

For *The Big X*, imagine heat or energy in the centre of the pelvis, radiating out to the ends of the hands and feet in the X, and then drawing everything into the centre in the folding action. This energy or heat flows out of the bones, and does not create or engage surface tension. In the second variation, imagine a direct line for the pathway of the initiating leg, not a circular action.

2) Rocking the Boat – Angels in the Snow

Gently slide the legs out along the floor. Begin to rock the body, initiating through the heel contact with the floor, allowing the head to nod "yes." Maintaining this easy rocking action, move the arms along the floor until they are directly above the head, and then back down again to the sides of the body, as if making snow angels with the arms only. After several repetitions, return to parallel stance.

IMAGERY

For *Rocking the Boat*, imagine the body floating in water, so that the rocking action is free of all tension, especially in the neck and upper back. Image the scapulae revolving in opposite directions like two wheels. Or, see the scapulae drawing the letter J and its mirror image, with the bottom loops going outward, away from the spine.

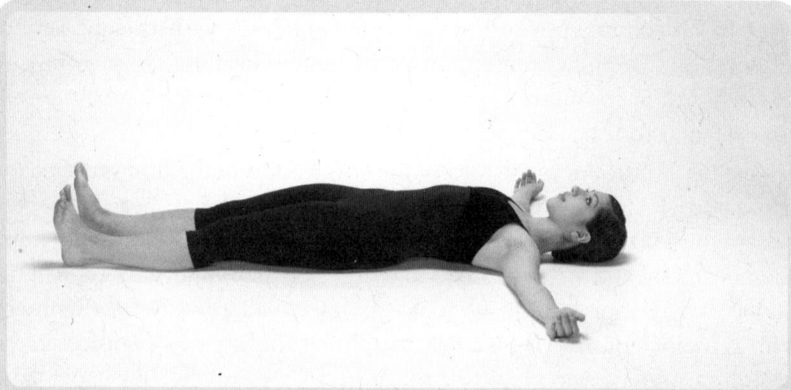

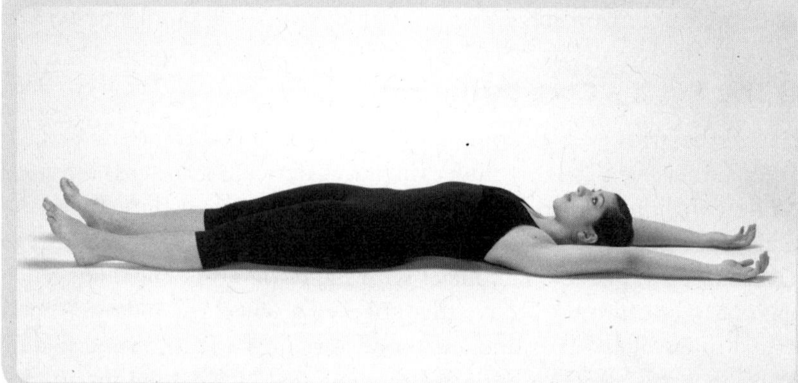

Notes for Teachers

Watch for excess effort and tension, especially in the neck and shoulders. Encourage the continued use of the breath rhythm and contact with the floor.

C – Gentle Warm-Up

Purpose

The purpose of this group of exercises is joint lubrication and blood flow to the muscles, essential areas of warm-up that should precede stronger activation of muscles (particularly in weight bearing) and increased range of motion. The rocking of the pelvis throughout *Rock and Stir* is also designed to lengthen the muscles of the lumbar spine, an area that is often tense in dancers. Continued attention to breath and whole body awareness will prepare the dancer for more complex activity to come. The use of sound in *Shake Out* (and later in the C-I Training work) is to inhibit tensing of the diaphragm, one of the contributors to core support. Tension and holding patterns in this important muscle can inhibit free use of breath.

1) Stretch Out

Begin lying supine, with the legs extended along the floor, arms by the sides of the body. Turn the palms to face the ceiling, and take the arms in a slow arc over the head along the floor. Inhale and stretch out in two directions, pointing the feet and reaching the arms. Exhale and sigh, relaxing all the limbs. Repeat the inhale and reaching action, this time with the feet and hands flexing (the toes point up to the ceiling and fingers point down to the floor). Exhale, sigh, and release again. Repeat once more, and on the last exhale, draw the legs all the way into the chest, wrapping the hands around the shins. Allow the full flexing of the thoracic and lumbar spine, leaving the head on the floor.

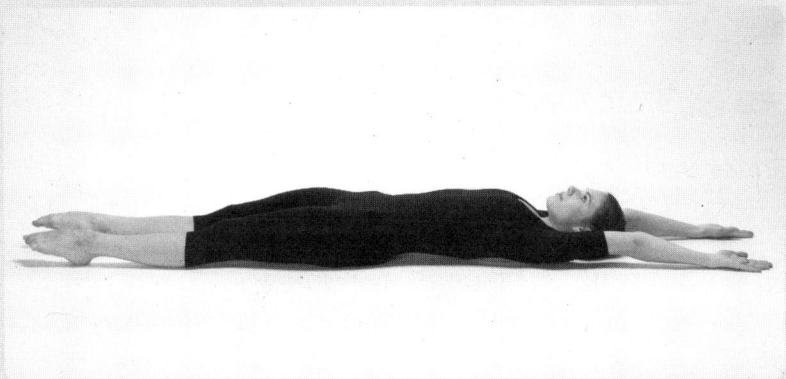

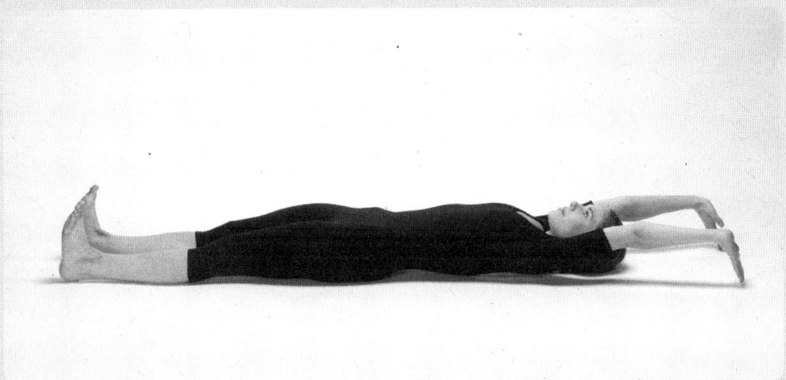

IMAGERY

For *Stretch Out*, imagine energy going out of the top of the head, and the ends of the fingers and toes (or wrists and heels in the variation using flexion), rather than tension and overuse of muscular effort. The reach should be an elongation of the entire spine and limbs. Imagine increasing the spaces between every bone and joint of the body.

2) Rock and Stir

Using the hands to move the legs, begin to rock the pelvis so that the legs come towards and away from the chest, the pelvis rocking off the floor. The spine will alternate between full lumbar flexion and neutral. Continuing this pelvic rocking action, begin to "stir the knees" in opposite directions, the legs mirroring each other with one leg moving clockwise and the other leg moving counter-clockwise. After several circles, reverse the direction. The action of stirring should be accomplished with no work in the leg muscles, but rather achieved entirely by the manipulation of the hands.

IMAGERY

For *Rock and Stir*, imagine the legs as two large spoons. The hands are holding the handles of the spoons, and stirring thick soup, so that the motion is very fluid and constant.

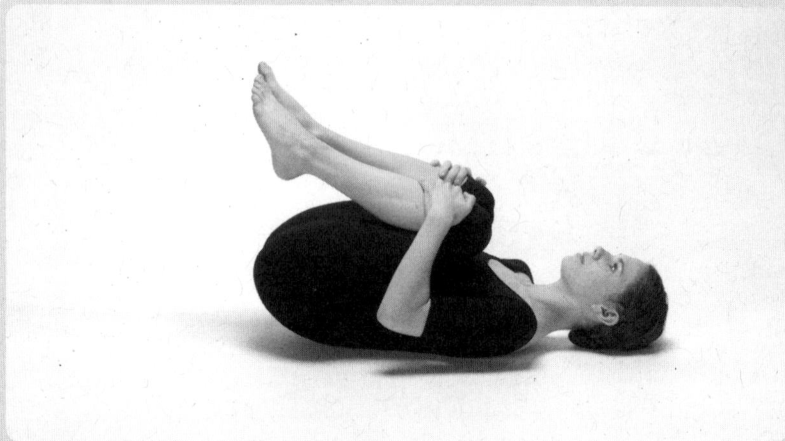

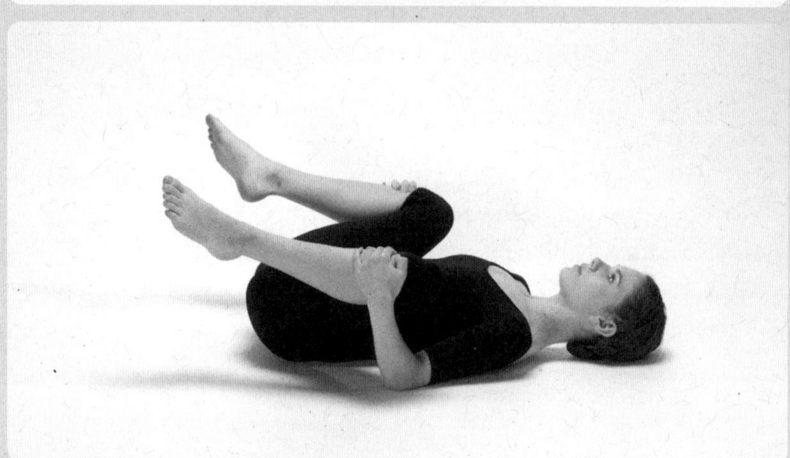

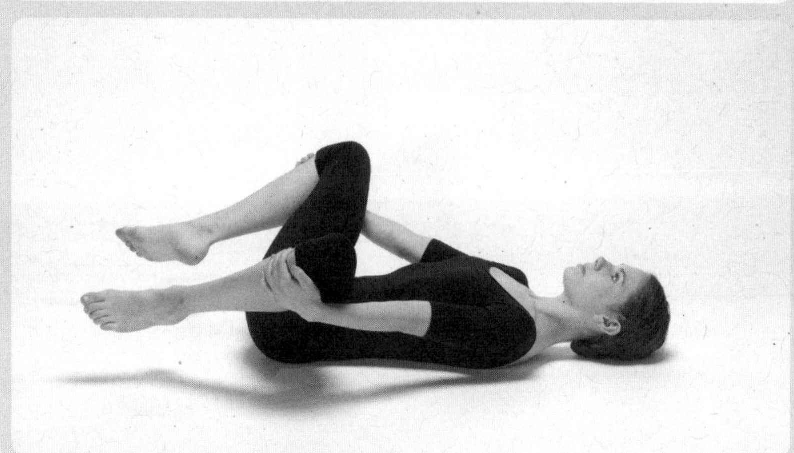

3) Shake Out

Take the arms and legs gently up to the ceiling. Rapidly shake and vibrate the arms and legs, making sure to mobilize all of the joints. Take a deep breath, and while vibrating, sound out. This should be a long, deep sound—an extended "Ahhhhh" from the diaphragm. Finish by leaving the legs "hanging in space" above the hips, knees, and feet (all soft), with the heels above the sitz bones, and the arms wrapped around the chest, as if hugging oneself.

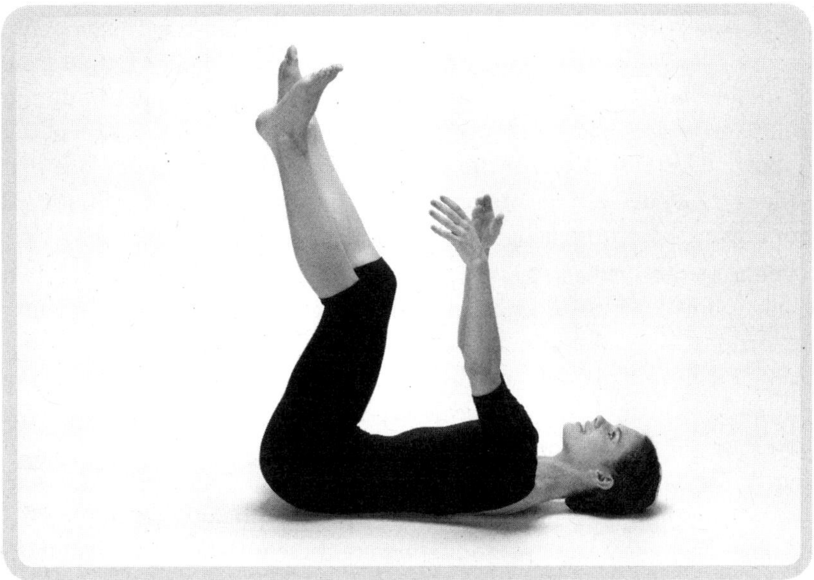

IMAGERY

For *Shake Out*, the action of shaking should be like a dog that gets out of a lake and tries to shake the water off.

Applications and Transfer to Standing and Travelling Work

In stance, the hips and lumbar spine are weight-bearing joints that handle high levels of compressive forces. For the long-term health of these joints, it is advisable to do some warm-up and gentle rhythmic motion prior to full weight bearing to ensure adequate lubrication. The stirring action is done passively, in terms of the muscles surrounding the hip joint, whereas once the body is in stance, the muscles must activate to resist the pull of gravity. Additionally, experiencing this articulation of the femur in the hip socket is crucial to standing and travelling legwork, especially leg extensions (développés).

Notes for Teachers

Remind the dancers about using little muscle effort, and to focus instead on the images and the bones. The quality of the sound in *Shake Out* can give the teacher information about whether the students are breathing freely or bracing and tightening the muscles around the rib cage that can interfere with easeful breathing. The sound should have a deep, rich quality as if it comes from deep in the belly, not high and tight in the throat.

D – Preparing the Feet and Ankles

Purpose

This group of exercises has many purposes. It is important to strengthen the muscles of the foot and ankle to correct or prevent foot pronation (rolling in)—a common alignment problem in dancers. The muscles targeted are the deep intrinsic arch muscles, the foot supinators (on the inside of the lower leg) pronators (on the outside of the lower leg), and the dorsiflexors of the ankle (on the front of the shin bones). Secondly, this series assists in organizing the alignment of the knee with the centre of the hip, and the foot with the knee. Thirdly, for the upper body, the arms are wrapped around the chest to relieve tension between the scapulae. This area between the shoulder blades is a common place that dancers hold excess tension, and this arm position has been modified from Sweigard's constructive rest position.

One of the primary causes of a range of injuries commonly called "shin splints" is muscle imbalance: weak dorsiflexors and tight plantar flexors, that is, weak in the front of the lower leg (shin) and tight in the back of the calf. This series can help prevent shin splints by strengthening the muscles at the front of the lower leg. (To address stretching tight posterior calf muscles, one can do lunges at the wall with both extended and flexed back knee, toes pointing forward or slightly turned in.) The muscles on the inside and outside of the foot (supinators and pronators) stabilize the ankle in relevé. Strengthening these muscles and learning to recruit them in good alignment may prevent ankle sprains.

1) Points and Squeezy Flexes

Start from the end of *Shake Out*, with the legs "hanging in space" above the hips, knees, and feet, which are all soft, with the heels above the sitz bones, and the arms wrapped around the chest, as if hugging oneself. Organize the legs so the hip, knee, and centre of the foot are in alignment. Point the feet sequentially through the heel, ball, and toe, in a rolling action on 1,2. On the reverse, however, instead of starting at the toes, squeeze the toes while pulling back to ankle dorsiflexion on 3, and only allow the toes to release into the extended position at the very end on 4. Do four to eight repetitions. Continue the foot action, adding a full extension of both legs on 1,2, and returning to the plié on 3,4. On the extension, the feet stay in line with the hip joints, reaching directly up to the ceiling. Do four to eight repetitions. The breath can exhale on the point/extend phase (1,2), and inhale on the flex/plié phase (3,4).

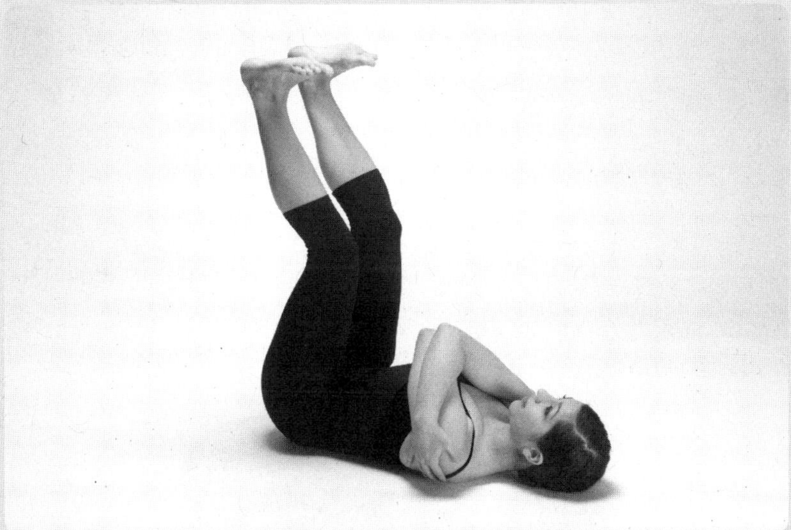

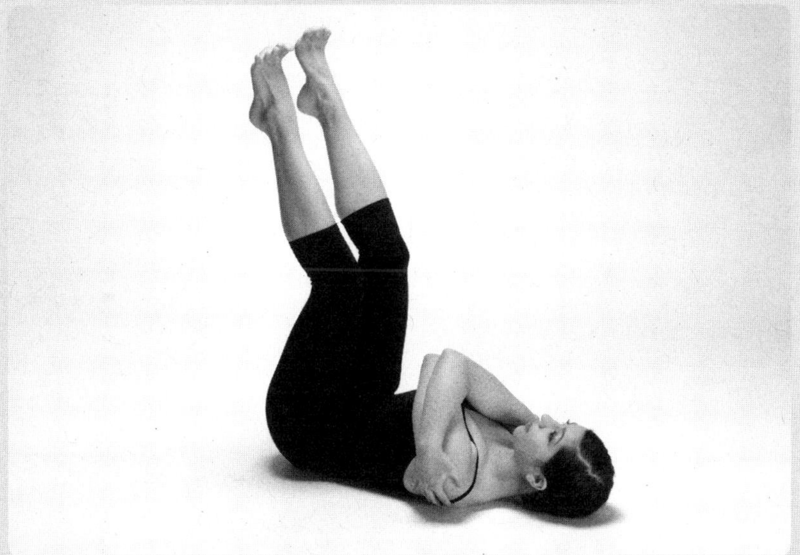

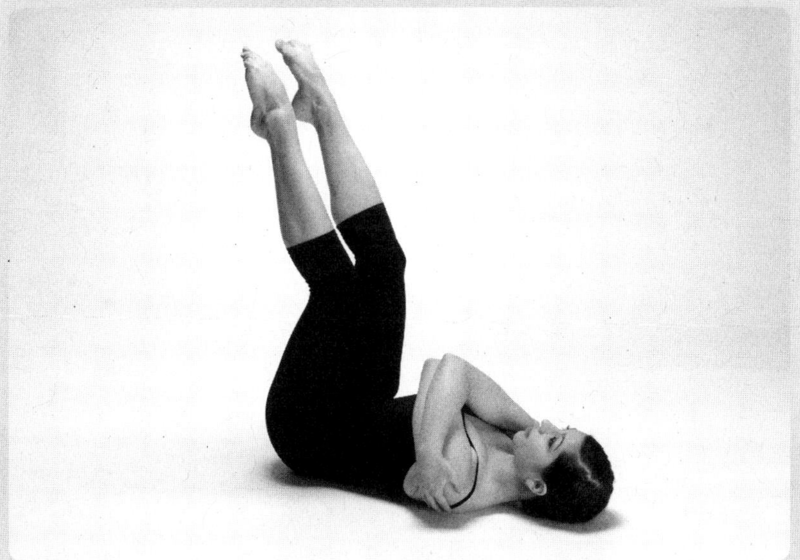

Photo Sequence continues on next page.

IMAGERY

For *Points and Squeezy Flexes*, imagine that the feet start flexed with pencils balanced across the feet at the junction of the toes to the metatarsal heads. As you point, push the pencils away, and, at the end of the movement, grab the pencils with the toes and pull them back towards you, releasing them back to the balance point. Additionally, imagine that each foot is moving in a narrow corridor, defined by the width of the knee joint. When adding the extension of the legs, imagine that the toes and feet are reaching higher in space, drawing the knees to the long position, as if the exhale of the breath is going out the ends of the toes. On the flex, the knees and ankles soften in response to gravity, with little muscle effort, other than that needed to maintain the parallel line of the legs and feet.

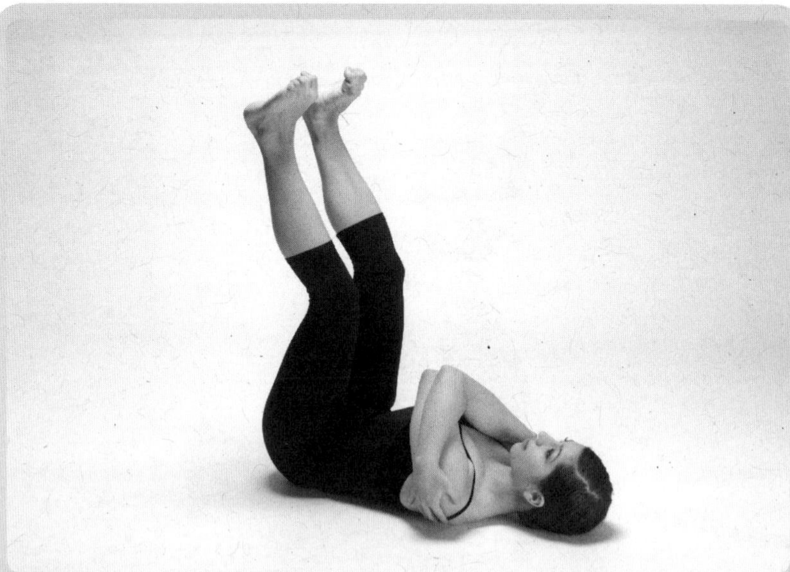

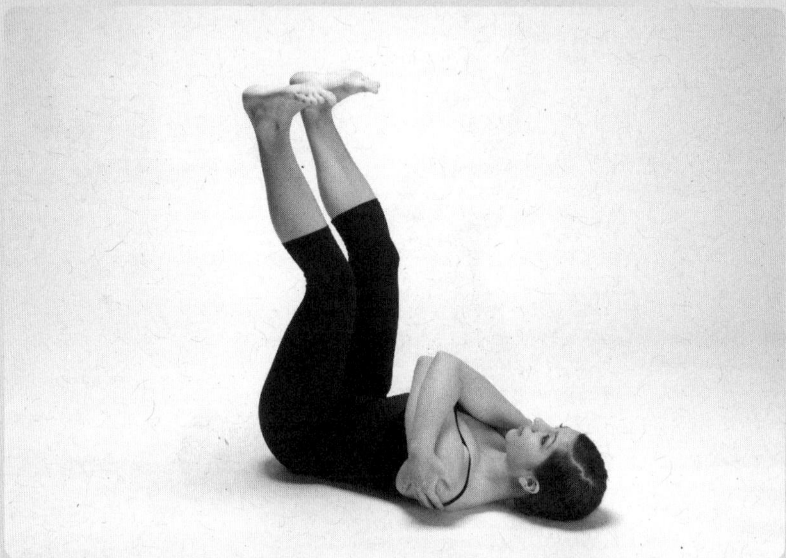

2) U-Shapes for the Ankles

This exercise also begins with the heels above the sitz bones, knees bent, and the arms wrapped around the chest, as if hugging oneself. Check that the hip, knee, and centre of the foot are in alignment. Now create the letter U with the feet, by circling them down and out on 1,2, and then down and in on 3,4. The exercise can be made more demanding by first spreading the toes on the outer part of the circle, and squeezing the toes on the inner part of the circle, and then reversing the toe action; that is, squeezing the toes on the outer part of the circle, and spreading the toes on the inner part of the circle. It is important that the thighs remain quiet and parallel, and that the action is isolated to the feet. If the dancer is having difficulty achieving this isolation, the hands can be placed inside the inner thighs, palms against the adductors, with a slight pressure pushing the legs open, and the legs resisting. Maintain the same breath rhythm as in *Points and Squeezy Flexes*.

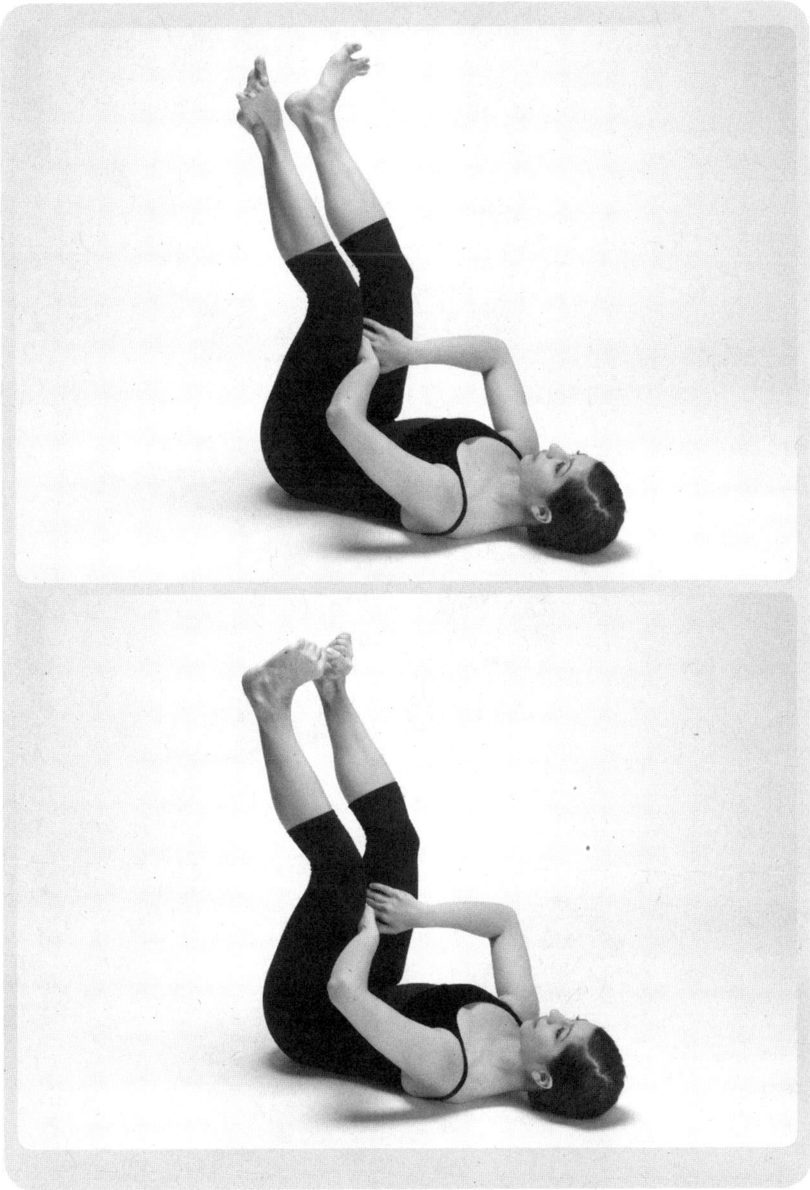

IMAGERY

For *U-Shapes for the Ankles*, the drawing of the letter U is primary. Once the hands are no longer needed on the inner thighs to maintain the parallel line, the dancer can imagine a tennis ball being squeezed between the knees.

3) Transition Back to Neutral Stance

There are two possible transitions from the end of *U-Shapes for the Ankles* to neutral parallel stance. One is to go to 90/90 (hip and knee joint both at 90° of flexion). Maintain the angle at the knee, keep the pelvis neutral, and return the feet slowly to the floor, continuing to breathe and soften the body surfaces. The more advanced version is to stretch the legs up, exhale as the legs are lowered to a 45° angle to the floor, and then bend the knees, lowering the feet to the floor, keeping the knees together. (Note: If the arms are still wrapped at the chest, leave them there for the start of the next series. If they have been placed between the inner thighs, bring the arms back across the chest.)

IMAGERY

For the transitions, imagine that the sacrum stays weighted on the floor to inhibit increased lumbar arch as the legs lower. Also, imagine the shoulders melting down towards the waistline as energy flows out of the top of the head.

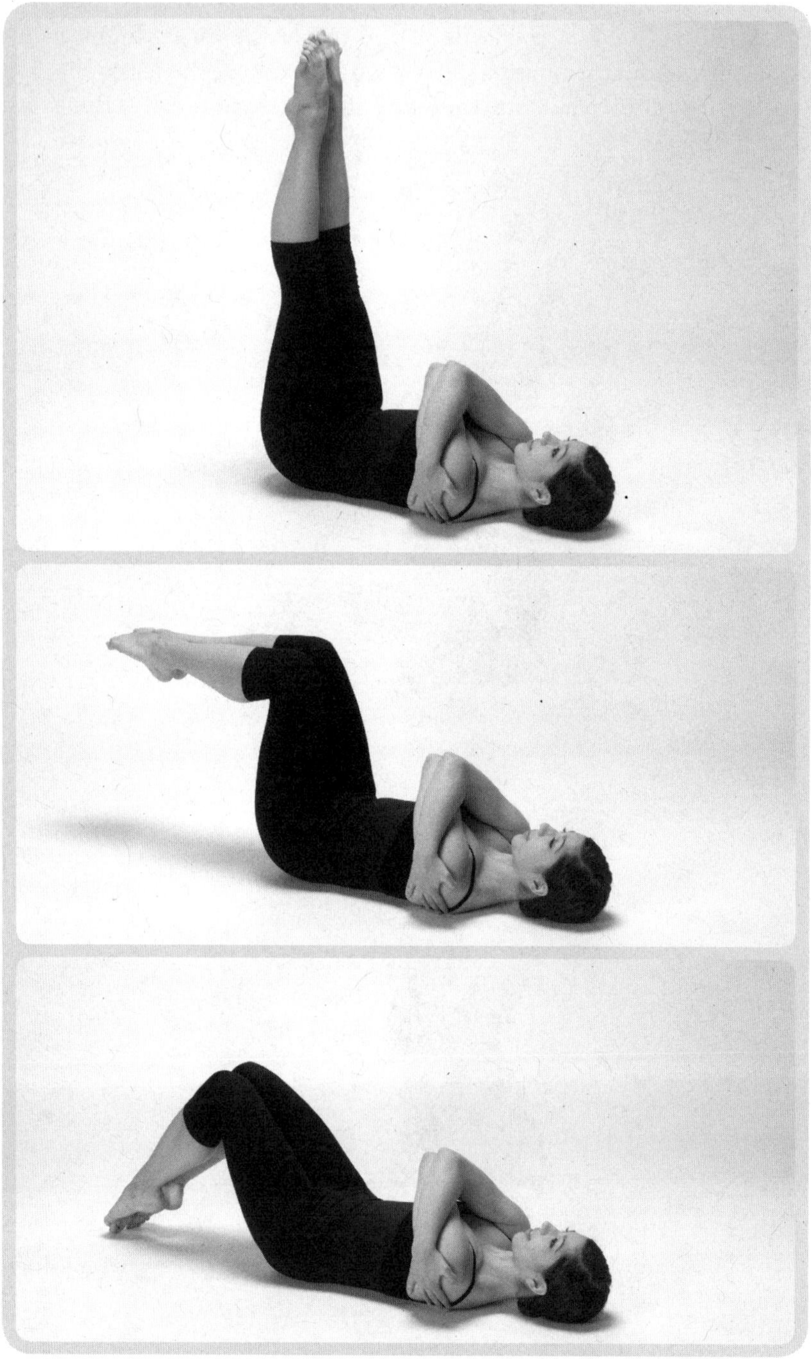

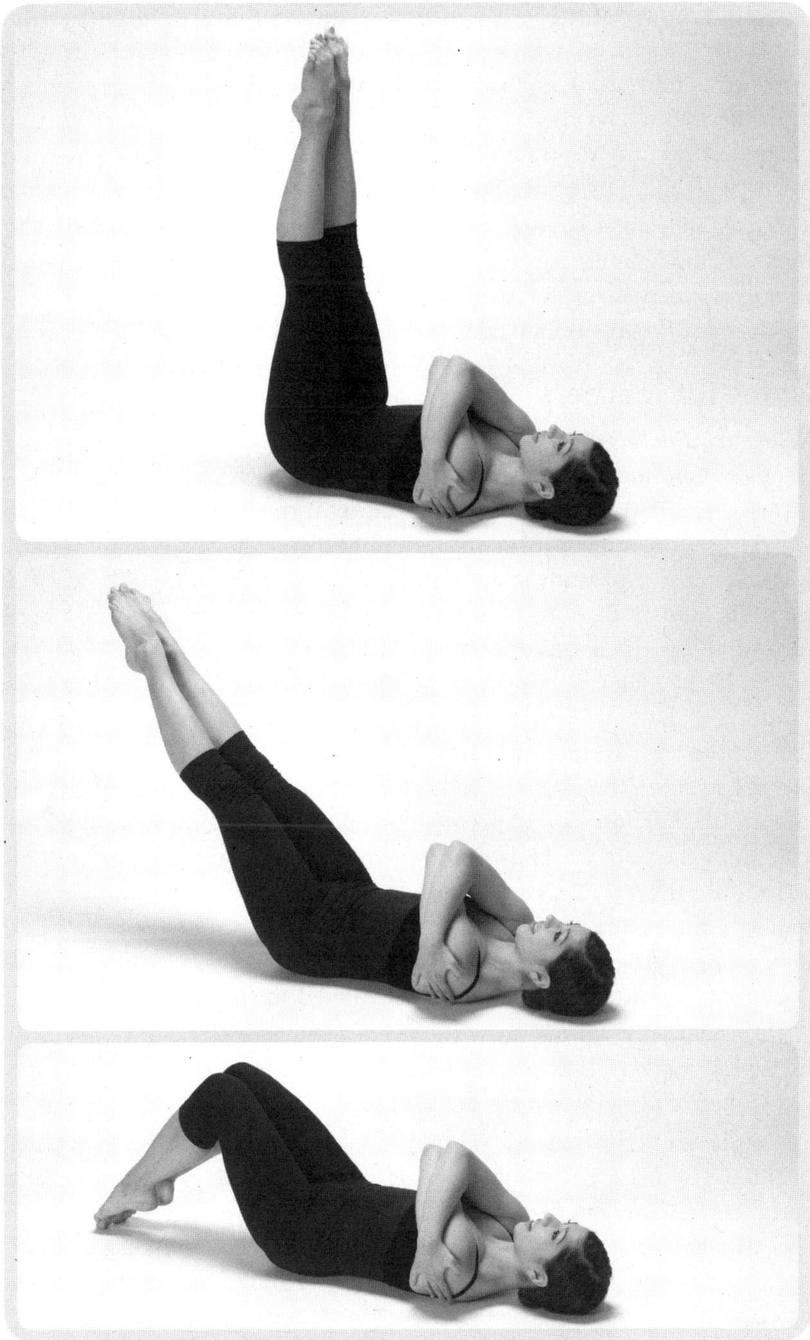

Applications and Transfer to Standing and Travelling Work

Along with images and awareness, this exercise series can assist with hip, knee, and foot organization in standing plié work. After doing the above exercises for the pronators and arches, stand in parallel first, that is, with the feet the width of the hip joints. Imagine water or sand coming out of the floor on the inside of the feet at the arches, pouring over the tops of the feet, and sinking into the floor by the fifth metatarsals. Roll gently to the inside and outside of the feet until you can arrive at the place where the weight is centred on the feet. Now turn out in first position, and demi plié. See a line or string dropping from the centre of the kneecap down to the part of the foot near the second toe. (Note: This image will not work for dancers with significant tibial torsion. A physical therapist or dance conditioning specialist will be able to provide specific guidance to dancers who have this twisting of the lower leg bones.) Use the image of the pelvis rising to straighten the legs and the knees (ankles softening to create the plié) bring awareness to the feet, and to the weight centring.

It is important to remember that in addition to these conditioning exercises, the habitual pattern of standing in pronation must be addressed through awareness, imagery, and an understanding of turnout support from the core and the hip joint, which will be discussed in detail in later sections.

Notes for Teachers

While dancers are doing the *Points and Squeezy Flexes*, make sure that the foot does not wing in and out, that the legs stay parallel, and that the centre of the foot lines up with the centre of the knee. Ideally, the heels should line up directly over the sitz bones, and the spine is in neutral. Many dancers will want to tuck under and press the low back into the floor in lumbar flexion. Continue to suggest the image of weighted sacrum and maintaining the natural lumbar curve to encourage neutral pelvis. If any dancers have so little range in the hamstrings that they cannot get the legs up over the hip joints without gripping in the hip flexor muscles, have them do one leg at a time, the other leg in neutral parallel stance. When using this modification, these dancers should not attempt the version extending the legs, but rather do one foot while the class does the first set, and the other foot as the class does the second set, adding the extensions. Regarding repetitions, begin with four and four, and then build up to eight and eight. Also recommended is a pause between the first and second sets, and the *U-Shapes for the Ankles* in the beginning. Eventually, these exercises can be done non-stop.

Regarding the crossed arms, people tend to have a favourite arm that they place on top. It is recommended that the dancers switch the top arm, when adding the extension of the legs.

Emphasize right from the beginning of this work to breathe, breathe, breathe! The breath rhythm, working slowly, and the use of awareness and imagery not only assists in decreasing the gripping of muscles, but also generally puts one into a parasympathetic state, which is a more receptive state for the brain in terms of repatterning. Indeed, the somatic practices are designed to bring the subject into a parasympathetic state, because it is believed that this is when change is possible on the noncon-scious level of muscle activation.

E – Patterning for the Arms

Purpose

For most dancers, this arm series does not enhance either strength or flex-ibility. Rather, it is for correct patterning (neural recruitment) of muscle groups for use of the arms in dance. Our goal in dance is to be able to reach the arms forward without the scapula abducting (protracting) and to take the arms over the head without the scapula elevating. The purpose of both variations in the *Port de Bras* exercise is to challenge the scapular and rib stabilization at a faster pace with more momentum and varying dynamics.

It should be noted that this exercise, and most of the exercises in the supine, neutral stance position, are done with the knees and feet together. The reason for this choice is the common muscle imbalance in dancers: tight and/or over-recruited lateral quadriceps (outer thighs) and weak and/or under-recruited adductors (inner thighs). Bringing the legs into closed neutral parallel stance is intended to compensate for this imbalance. Additionally, for both beginning dancers and trained dancers who have habitually worked in forced turn out (that is, trying to stand in 180° at the feet when this is beyond the rotation allowed by the hip joint), in open parallel stance the feet will tend to drift away from parallel. Keeping the knees and feet touching will help maintain the parallel line of the feet, and give the dancer kinesthetic feedback about this position.

1) Arm Series on 8

Begin in parallel stance as described above, with the arms crossed at the chest. Unfold the arms into a large oval directly above the rib cage, in line with the bottom of the sternum. On count 1, extend the arms fully towards the ceiling and spread the hands and fingers, palms facing each other, allowing the shoulder blades to come up off the floor. (Note an acceptable variation: For some individuals, the full use of the arms can cause the back of the neck to shorten, and a slight backward tilt of the head.) On count 2, widen the scapulae onto the floor, elongating the back of the neck, and returning the arms to the oval. Think of the upper back staying wide during this action. On count 3, widen the arms out to the sides, into what would be considered a classical second position, maintaining the round shape of the entire arm, with no part of the arm touching the floor. On count 4, return to the oval over the rib cage, keeping the front of the chest very wide. Repeat counts 1 and 2, for counts 5 and 6. On count 7, move the arms up to high fifth position above the head, again keeping the arms round, and off the floor, and the back of the rib cage on the floor. On count 8, return to the oval once more, to start the series over. Complete four sets, ending the last one in high fifth position.

Breath rhythm: Begin the series with the exhale, and continue exhaling on all the odd counts, inhaling on the even counts.

Photographs of the *Arm Series on 8* can be found on pages 20–21.

IMAGERY

As the arms reach up, imagine that the space between the scapulae widens and expands, and as the shoulders return to the floor, maintain this width in the back as the chest opens and expands in the front.

Imagine that energy continues to pour out of the top of the head for the whole series, releasing and elongating the back of the neck, without muscular effort.

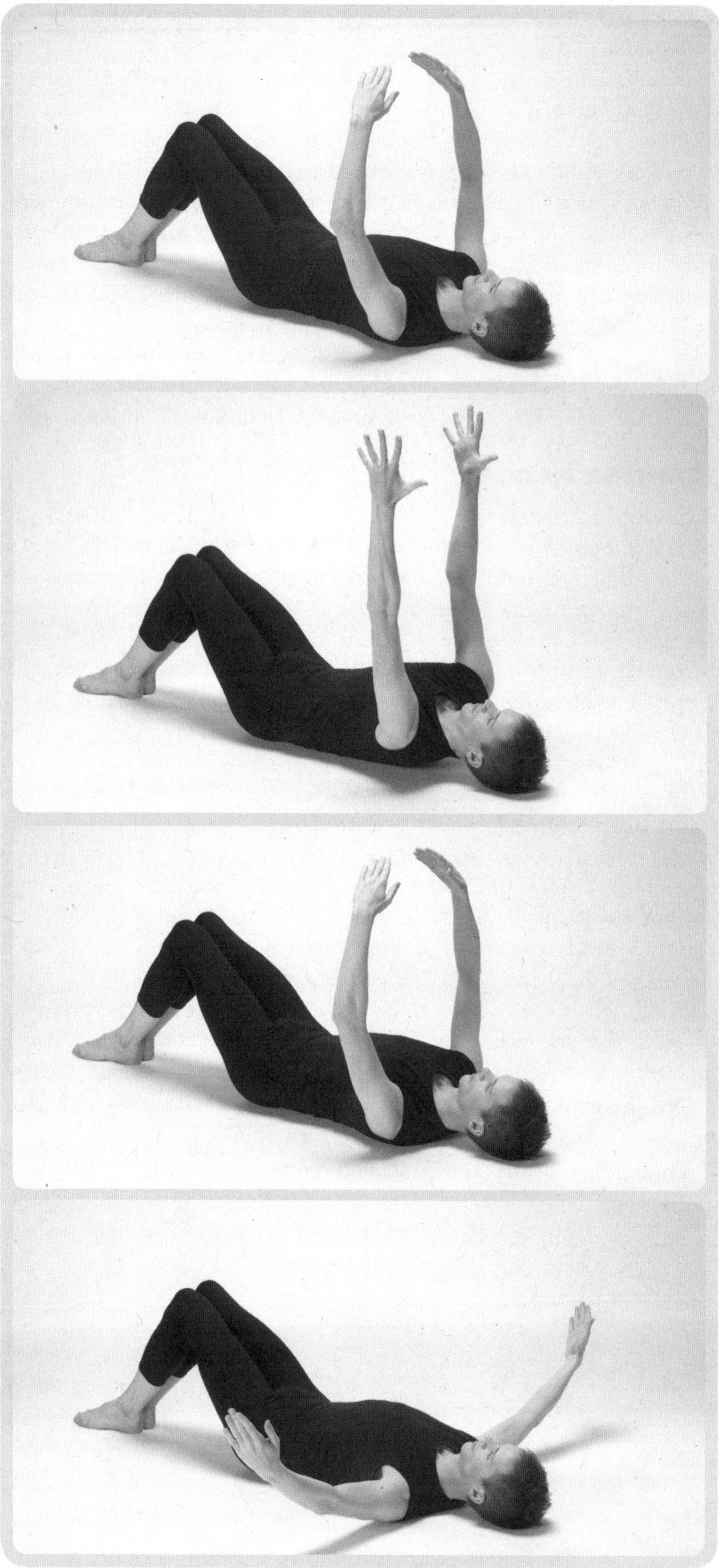

IMAGERY

As the arms are lifting up to fifth position, image the rib cage becoming very soft, and sinking into the floor, especially the sides and bottom of the rib cage. At the same time, the scapulae melt down towards the waist, and the distance between the shoulders and the ears elongates.

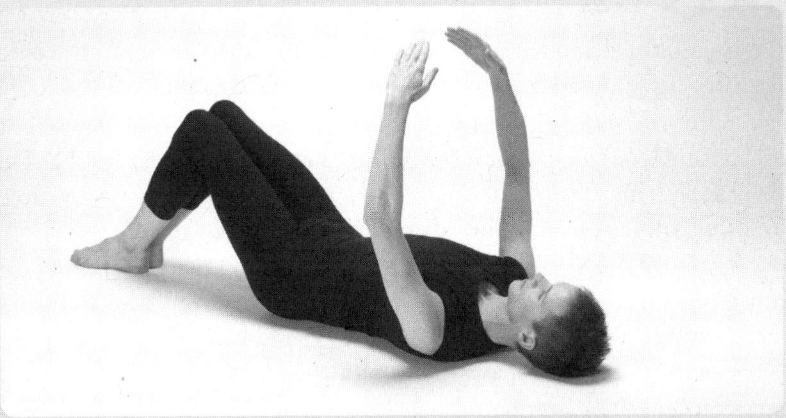

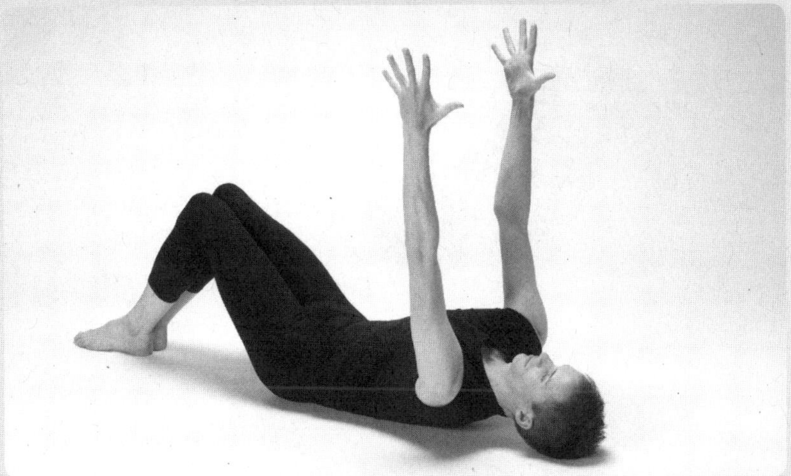

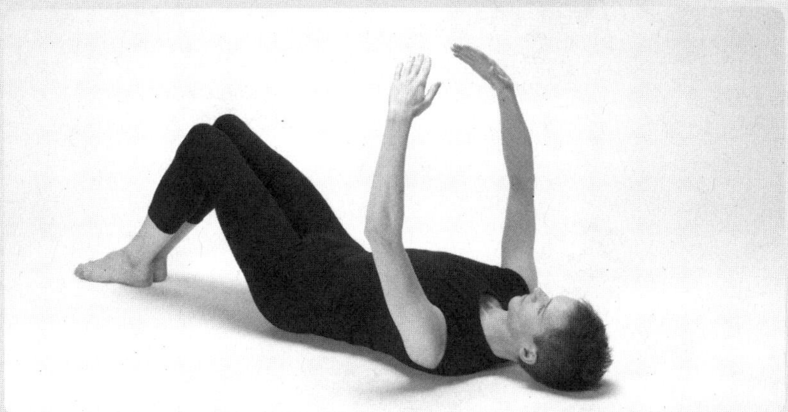

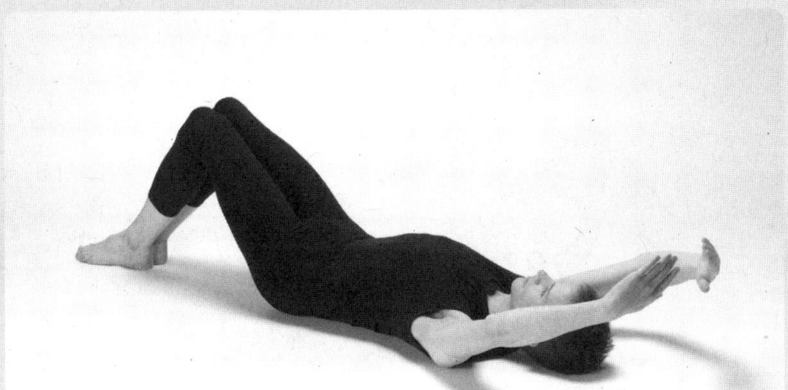

IMAGERY

Imagine creating large volumes of space between the arms in each position, as if one is holding a large ball in front of or above the body.

To maintain the connection of the inner thighs throughout the series, imagine that there is a thin sheet of paper or glass between the knees and inner thighs that must be held in place. This image will reoccur in later legwork, so it is useful to establish it at this point in the arm series.

2) Port de Bras

These should be done at a faster pace than the *Arm Series on 8*, eventually working up to a very fast rhythm. There are two possible variations.

Variation 1 – Classical port de bras, going in both directions: From fifth position going to second position, down to bras bas, and back up to fifth position, four times, and then reversing direction four times, finishing with alternating directions.

Variation 2 – Successional port de bras, going in both directions: From fifth position going to second position and returning to fifth position, but in this variation, allowing the arms to cross at the chest staying close to the body, rather than passing through the open oval, four times each direction, and then alternating.

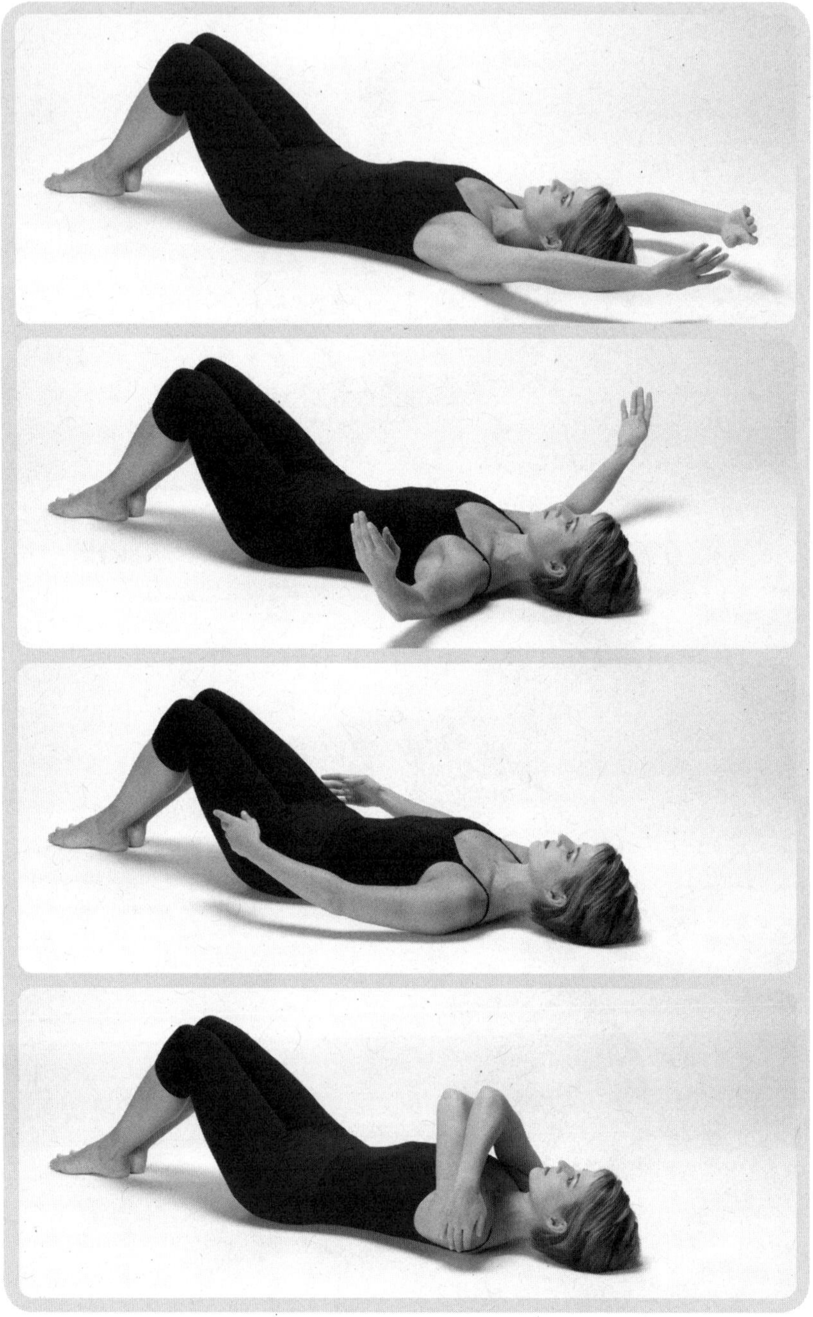

Applications and Transfer to Standing and Travelling Work

This work directly transfers to arm movements in stance and travelling work in class. The same images can be suggested (soft ribs, embracing volumes, wide back and chest) once the dancer is up off the floor.

Notes for Teachers

It is useful, when first teaching this series, to describe to the dancers the movements of the scapulae, the movements of the arm in the shoulder joint, and how these movements organize in daily life. Then explain how we change these patterns for dance aesthetics. Sometimes teachers use language that gives dancers the impression that the shoulder blades are completely static and immobilized during movements of the arms in dance. It is important for the dancers to understand and allow the rotary action the scapulae make when the arms go overhead. An image that can be used in standing work is that the scapulae are wheels that are attached at their hubs (centres) to the rib cage. The wheels can revolve in both directions, but the hubs of the wheels do not drift up and down or side to side.

Some dancers will raise the arms too high when opening out to second, and end up with hands that would be above shoulder height in stance. If the dancer cannot correctly sense this placement, they can visually look to the side, or work with partners for assistance. Also, dancers can be reminded that the palms face the ceiling in second, and the head in fifth. Note that if the dancer cannot keep the ribs dropped on the floor as the arms rise to fifth, it may be due to tightness in the pectoralis minor muscle in the chest. Stretches for this muscle will be addressed later. In the meantime, the dancer should minimize the range of motion, maintaining quiet ribs.

F – Introducing Core Support

Purpose

The purpose of this series is first and foremost to introduce the concept and experience of narrowing and hollowing for core support. Many dancers rely on the surface muscles (rectus abdominus), and tighten or brace these muscles to feel stable. However, the deeper muscles are more critical for core support for a number of reasons: (1) they can be recruited in any and all movements of the spine; (2) they are tonic rather than phasic, meaning they function in a continuous action rather than in short bursts; (3) research indicates that they anticipate weight being loaded onto the torso (such as partnering work), and are thus extremely important for injury prevention; and (4) from an aesthetic perspective, they create the lifted look dancers want to achieve, rather than compressing the torso and creating a bulge in abdominal crunches.

After narrowing and hollowing is established, it is important that the dancer learn how to achieve this action with all possible movements of the spine, both for stability and balance, and for injury prevention. The *Undercurves and Overcurves* should always be done with a focus on narrowing and hollowing as the foundation for these movements. The *Small Curls* and *Small Curls with a Twist* begin to develop increased strength in the obliques and rectus abdominus, but should also be approached with *Narrowing and Hollowing* as the basis.

The following series establishes a foundation for all of the later abdominal exercises. The first of these, *Narrowing and Hollowing*, should be integrated into all the abdominal work and legwork throughout the C-I Training system.

1) Narrowing and Hollowing

While exhaling, imagine a narrowing of the waist, and a sinking or hollowing in the front of the pelvis. This is the action of the deepest abdominal muscle, the transverse abdominus. There will be a subtle sensation of the waist and front of the body drawing or collecting inward. This muscle does not significantly flex or extend the spine, so the drawing action should be accomplished without visible movement of the pelvis. Additionally, there should be no tightening or bracing of the surface abdominal muscles (rectus abdominus), and the surface should remain supple. Do several repetitions until this can be accomplished easily.

IMAGERY

For *Narrowing and Hollowing*, imagine that an energy or magnet is drawing the waist and front of the pelvis in towards the spine at the same time that a belt at the waist is shrinking. It can also be useful to imagine that the torso is a big tube of toothpaste and that as the tube is squeezed in the centre, toothpaste shoots out the top of the head and the bottom of the pelvis.

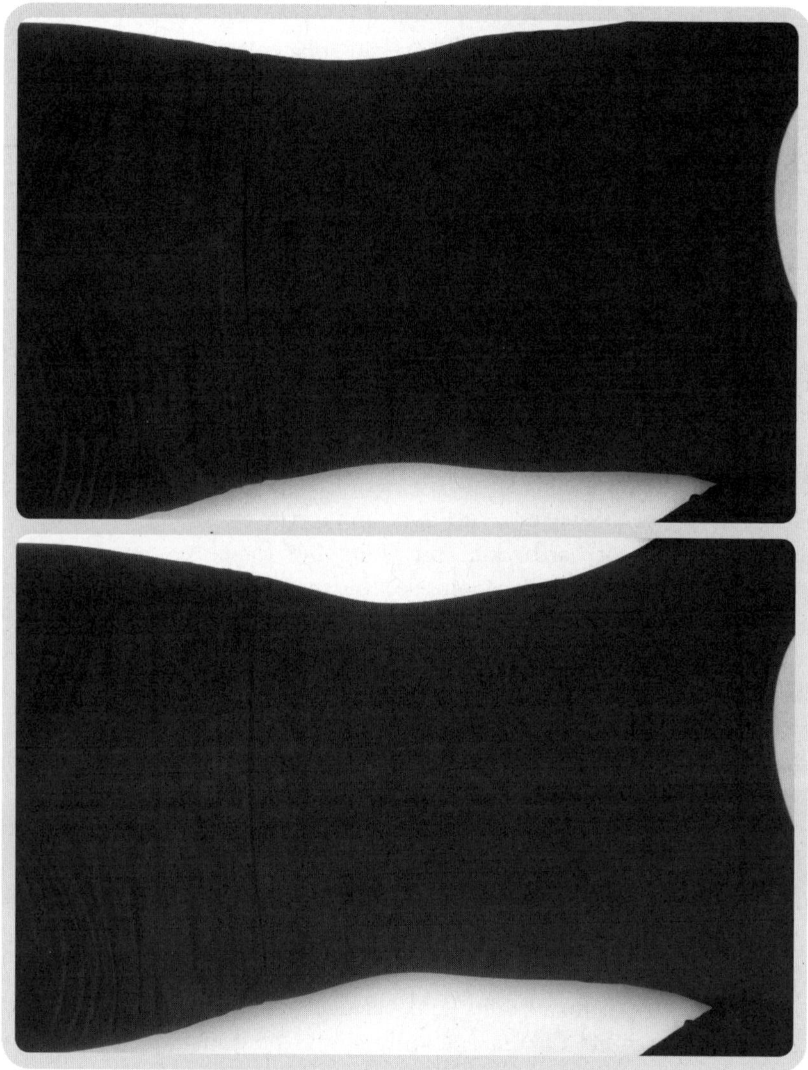

2) Undercurves

The next stage is to learn to recruit this deep muscle during spine action. Begin by exhaling, narrowing and hollowing, and then immediately roll the pelvis into posterior tilt, or full lumbar flexion on 1,2. This movement is called the undercurve. Be aware of the sacrum maintaining contact with the floor, and keeping the focus of muscle action on the abdominals, rather than squeezing or pushing with the gluteus maximus. After the spine flexion action, return the pelvis to neutral each time on 3,4, inhaling to prepare for the next undercurve. Do eight or more repetitions.

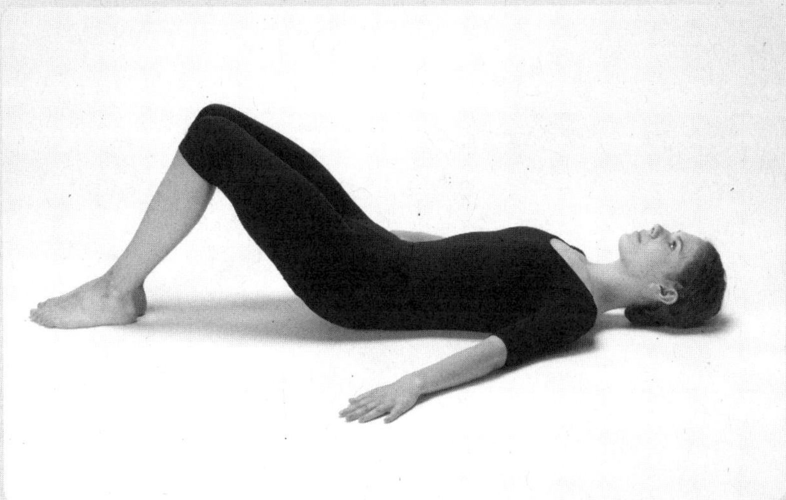

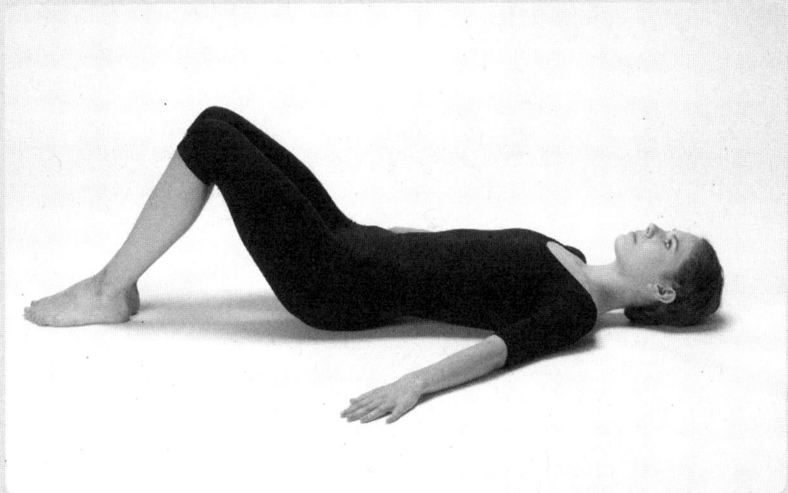

IMAGERY

For *Undercurves*, imagine a row of elastic bands that line up along the pubic bone and run up along the body towards the navel. In the mind's eye, gather the top end of these elastics into a group, so that the elastics now form a triangle. Drop this top point of the triangle to the place on the lumbar spine directly underneath the navel. On the undercurve, the elastics shorten to draw the pubic bone towards the lumbar spine. Or, try to see a giant ice cream scooper that starts at the pubic bone and scoops out a big ball of ice cream as it moves up the body towards the navel. A third image is to imagine two huge paddlewheels (like those on the steamboats on the Mississippi River) attached to the sides of the pelvis, at the ilium on each side. On the undercurve, imagine the wheels rotating towards the upper body. On the return to neutral, the wheels revolve in the opposite direction.

3) Undercurves and Overcurves

When the undercurve has been achieved, add the remainder of range of motion in flexion/extension of the lumbar spine. From the undercurve on 1,2, go beyond neutral pelvis to the overcurve on 3,4, a full arching of the lumbar spine, but maintaining the hollowing throughout, so that the abdominals (front of the pelvis) do not bulge outward. Do eight or more repetitions, at a slightly slower tempo than #2 above. If the breathing becomes forced or is held, sounding and vocalization can assist in keeping the breathing natural, creating the sound "Huh" in a low pitch on the exhale/undercurve.

IMAGERY

For *Undercurves and Overcurves*, the elastics shorten on the undercurve and lengthen, but remain taut, on the overcurve, providing a support for the front of the abdominals. The paddlewheels can also be used for the overcurves, rolling the wheels further to go beyond neutral. Another useful image is that the spine is like a slinky and in the overcurve, the spaces between the vertebrae expand in the front of the spine, rather than compress in the posterior spine, and the two ends of the slinky (at the bottom of the ribs and the tailbone) do not move closer together.

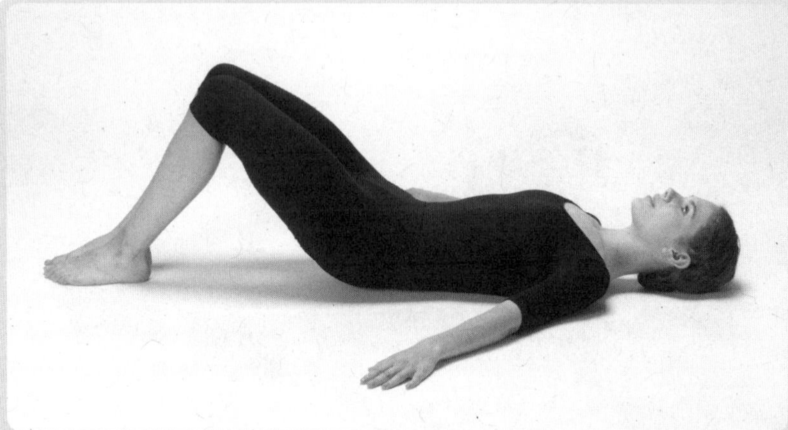

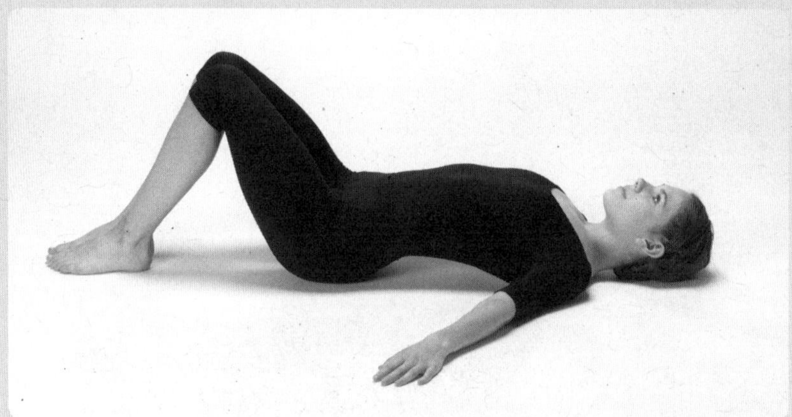

4) Preparations for Small Curls

Finish *Undercurves and Overcurves* in a full undercurve of the pelvis. Bring the head and shoulders up off the floor, softening the sternum into the back and maintaining a space under the chin. Reach the arms forward and take hold of the hamstrings close to the knee joints. In this position, called the *Bowl of the Body*, the arms are long, the head and knees are at approximately the same height, and the spine is rounded. Ideally, the top of the head points to the ceiling. Inhale, and then slowly exhale, deeply narrowing and hollowing, and observing the sinking of the abdominals towards the floor. Repeat four times. Release the hands from holding the legs and repeat. The arms are soft and round, but reaching out past the thighs, parallel to the floor. Repeat the breathing and sinking. Slowly lower down and return to neutral pelvis.

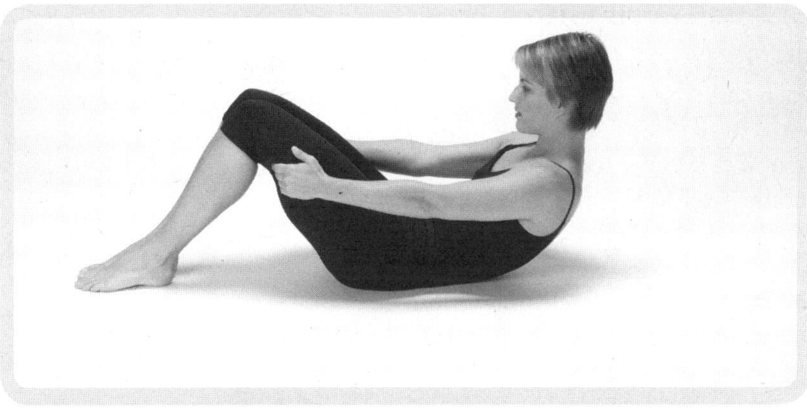

IMAGERY

For the *Preparations for Small Curls*, imagine that the bowl deepens and widens with each exhale. The bowl is a three-dimensional image, and curves in every plane. The image of the ice cream scooper can also be used for this exercise. See the shoulders widening in the back, but also melting down towards the waist.

5) Small Curls

From the end of *Undercurves and Overcurves*, finish in a full undercurve of the pelvis. Bring the head and shoulders up off the floor, softening the sternum into the back, and maintaining a space under the chin. The arms are soft and round, but reaching out past the thighs, parallel to the floor. Ideally, the top of the head points to the ceiling. On the exhale, sink the abdominals more deeply into the floor, curling the body up higher on 1. The sacrum should stay on the floor, and each small curl should deepen the sensation of hollowing and rounding. Again, the "Huh" sound on the curl can keep the breathing free. On 2, lower only as far as the starting position for this exercise (the *Bowl of the Body*), not all the way down to the floor. Do eight to sixteen repetitions. Finish in the last lift, exhale two to three times with increased hollowing, and then slowly lower down and return to neutral pelvis.

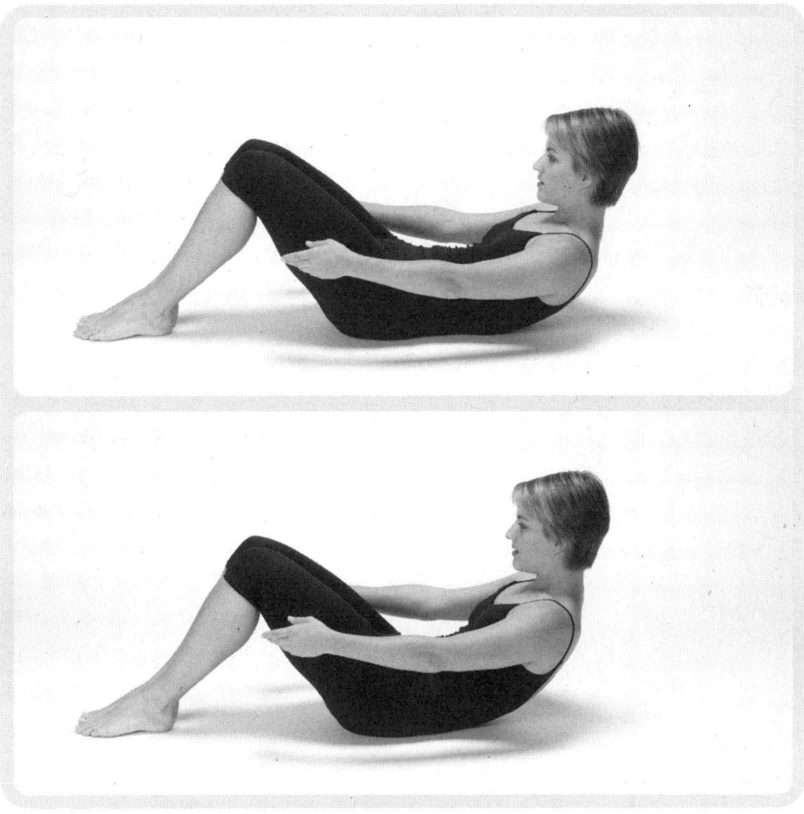

IMAGERY

For *Small Curls*, imagine that with each lift, the abdominals sink more into the floor. Another image is a hand on the abdominals gently pressing them down as the body curls up.

6) Small Curls with a Twist

Do the same action, breathing, and vocalization as in *Small Curls*, but each time the body lifts, add a twist, alternating sides. Both arms should cross over to one side of the thighs. Make sure that there is no jerking action or momentum used to lift the body, but rather the pressing down of the deep abdominals, and a slow and smooth lifting of the upper spine. Alternate eight plain curls, eight with a twist, and repeat. Do one last lift in the centre, exhale two to three times with increased hollowing, and then slowly lower down and return to neutral pelvis.

IMAGERY

For *Small Curls with a Twist*, imagine the shoulder being drawn towards the opposite hip on the curl up with the twist.

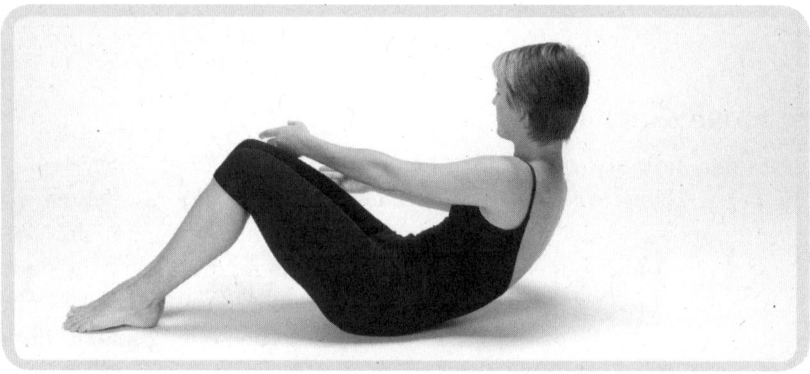

7) Advanced Variation

Small Curls and *Small Curls with a Twist* can be done with the feet off the floor, lower legs parallel to the floor, inner thighs together. Legs should remain quiet.

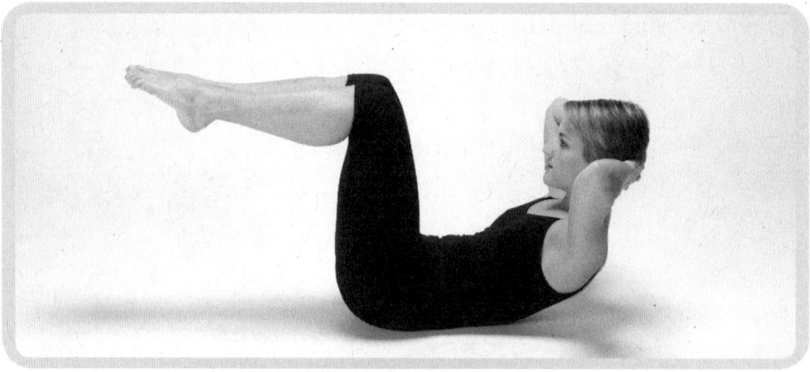

Applications and Transfer to Standing and Travelling Work

The use of narrowing and hollowing applies directly to dance positions and movements such as arabesque, leaps, port de corps, and in modern dance, all of the off-centre work. The overcurve is especially important, to support all the work in dance with the spine arched. The image of the elastic bands can be used in stance to shift the positioning of the pelvis. If the dancer is standing in anterior tilt (swayback), the elastics can be shortened; if the dancer is in posterior tilt (tucked), the elastics can be lengthened. The image of the toothpaste tube will assist in establishing narrowing and hollowing in stance, while making the body taller. Terminology such as "lift up" or "pull up" can sometimes create distortions of the alignment, such as forward and overlifted ribs. Images that create length of the entire spine from internal sensations are helpful in creating lift in good alignment.

Notes for Teachers

There is some disagreement currently as to whether it is best to exhale or inhale on the narrowing and hollowing action. Probably the best advice is to make sure that the dancers are not holding their breath, and that the breathing is natural and not forced. Eventually, while dancing, the deep core support muscles must be recruited during the full cycle of inhaling and exhaling, and hence should be learned in whatever pattern is easiest for the dancer and then attempted throughout the cycle. It is useful to encourage the dancers to look at the abdominals during the *Small Curls* and *Small Curls with a Twist*, and to "see" these muscles sinking towards the floor. This visual feedback reinforces the sensory learning. Note: For the entire curl series, the upper back (both scapulae) remains off the floor. Each curl takes the body higher than this starting position. To find the starting position of the spine for *Small Curls*, it can be useful to repeat the preparation on the day that *Small Curls* are introduced; that is, come up to the point where the hands are holding the hamstrings close to the knee joints and the spine is fully curved, with lumbar spine on the floor, but not the upper spine. Release the hands from the backs of the legs. This is the lowest part of the curl.

G – Mobilizing the Upper Torso

Purpose

The primary purpose of this series is to mobilize the shoulder joint for range of motion. For dancers, it is desirable to have free movement of the arms without unnecessary movement of the shoulder blades and spine, just as it is desirable to have lower limb movement without unnecessary movement of the pelvis. Secondly, it is designed to release the tension dancers carry in the rhomboids, the muscles that connect the scapulae to the spine and inhibit the shoulders from rounding forward during arm gestures. This is why it is important to allow the scapulae to move away from the spine in the forward reach. Thirdly, this series aids in stretching out the posterior hip muscles due to the inward rotation of the bent leg during *The Clock* and the stretch afterwards. Fourthly, by allowing the chest to roll towards and away from the floor, there is an important rotary component for the spine in non-weight bearing. This action will assist in lubricating the articular facets of the spine, and potentially delay wear and tear on these important joints. Most dance forms incorporate considerable spine rotation (ballet arabesque and épaulement, modern dance, jazz and ballroom spirals, and so on), and warming up the facets in non-weight bearing can be beneficial for good joint health. The stretching phases release tension in the pectoralis major (*First Spiral Stretch*) and the pectoralis minor (*Second Spiral Stretch*); tension in these muscle groups can cause rounded shoulders in dancers. The pectoralis minor is particularly important because if it is tight, it will pull the ribs forward when the dancer attempts to open and align the shoulders. Finally, the roll back to the sacrum engages the oblique abdominals due to the recruitment of these muscles from a spiraled position.

1) Preparation

Starting from parallel stance, point the right foot so that the big toe touches the floor, and the ankle comes into alignment with the tibia (shin bone). Bring the thigh towards the chest, remembering to maintain the sacrum connection to the floor so that the pelvis does not tuck under. Take hold of the leg by interlocking the fingers of both hands around the shin just under the knee joint. Now take the attention to the left leg and flex the left foot. On the exhale, slide the left leg out along the floor, reaching out the heel and top of the head. Point the left foot successionally; that is, start at the heel, then the metatarsus (ball of the foot), and finish reaching out the toes. Gently release the right leg across the body, guiding it with the left hand and allowing the pelvis to roll in that direction until the right knee and foot are placed on the floor on the left side of the body. At the same time, open the right arm out to the side in line with the shoulder, allowing the upper torso to open towards the ceiling, and turn the focus to the right hand, palm up. The arm may or may not touch the floor. The left leg, knee, and foot can now relax and soften.

IMAGERY

For *Preparation*, imagine the fold or crease at the hip joint deepening and sinking during the hip flexion (as the thigh is moving towards the chest). As the heel of the lower leg slides out, imagine that breath or energy or light is flowing out the heel and top of the head in opposite directions and the waist is narrowing. The tube of toothpaste image can also be suggested. As the right leg moves across the body to the floor, imagine gravity moving the leg with as little effort as possible.

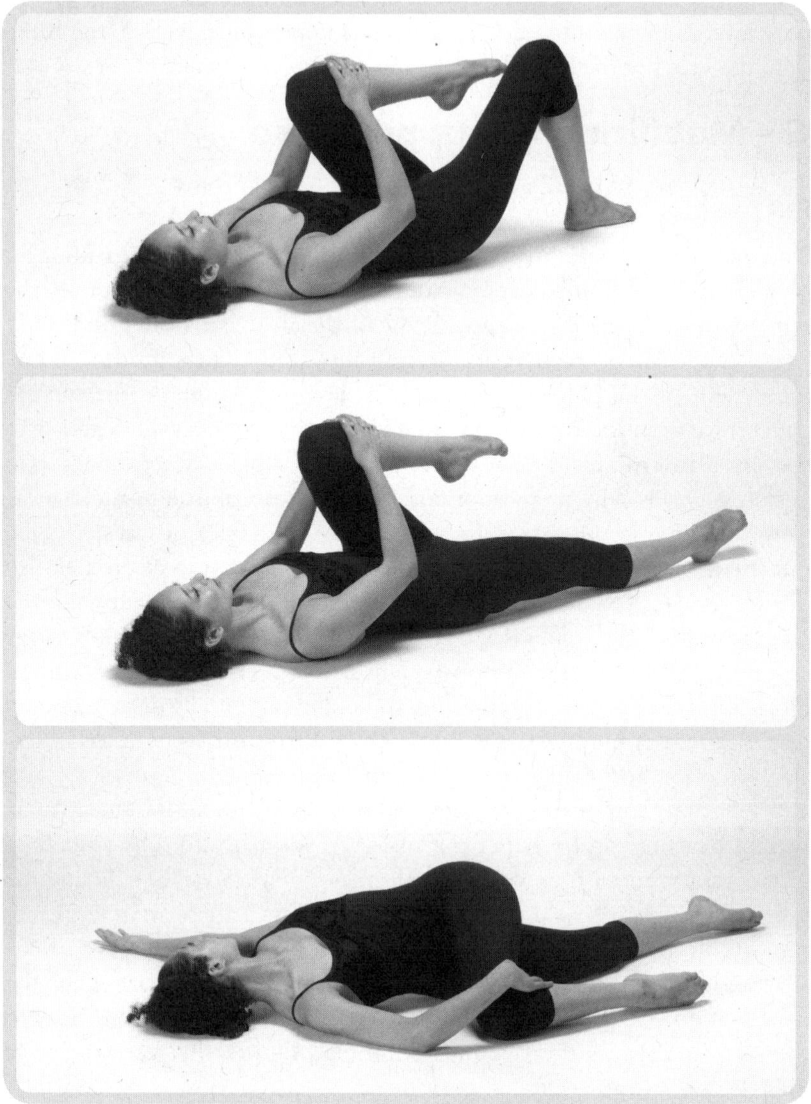

2) The Clock

Imagine the body lying in the centre of a huge clock. The right hand is reaching towards nine o'clock, palm facing up to the ceiling. Slowly move the arm in a large circle, keeping it as close to the floor as comfortable, until the hand is reaching to twelve o'clock on count 1, then to three o'clock on count 2 (palm now facing down to the floor), down to six o'clock on count 3, and back to nine o'clock by count 4. The focus should follow the hand, and the upper torso should be allowed to roll with the arm movement, so that on 2 the chest faces the floor and on count 4 the chest faces the ceiling. The neck and shoulders remain as relaxed as possible, and the pelvis remains fairly quiet, not rotating to face the floor and ceiling with the chest. (Note: As the hand reaches to three o'clock and the chest rolls to face the floor, the scapula should move away from the spine, allowing for full range. Do four repetitions, then reverse direction and do four repetitions.)

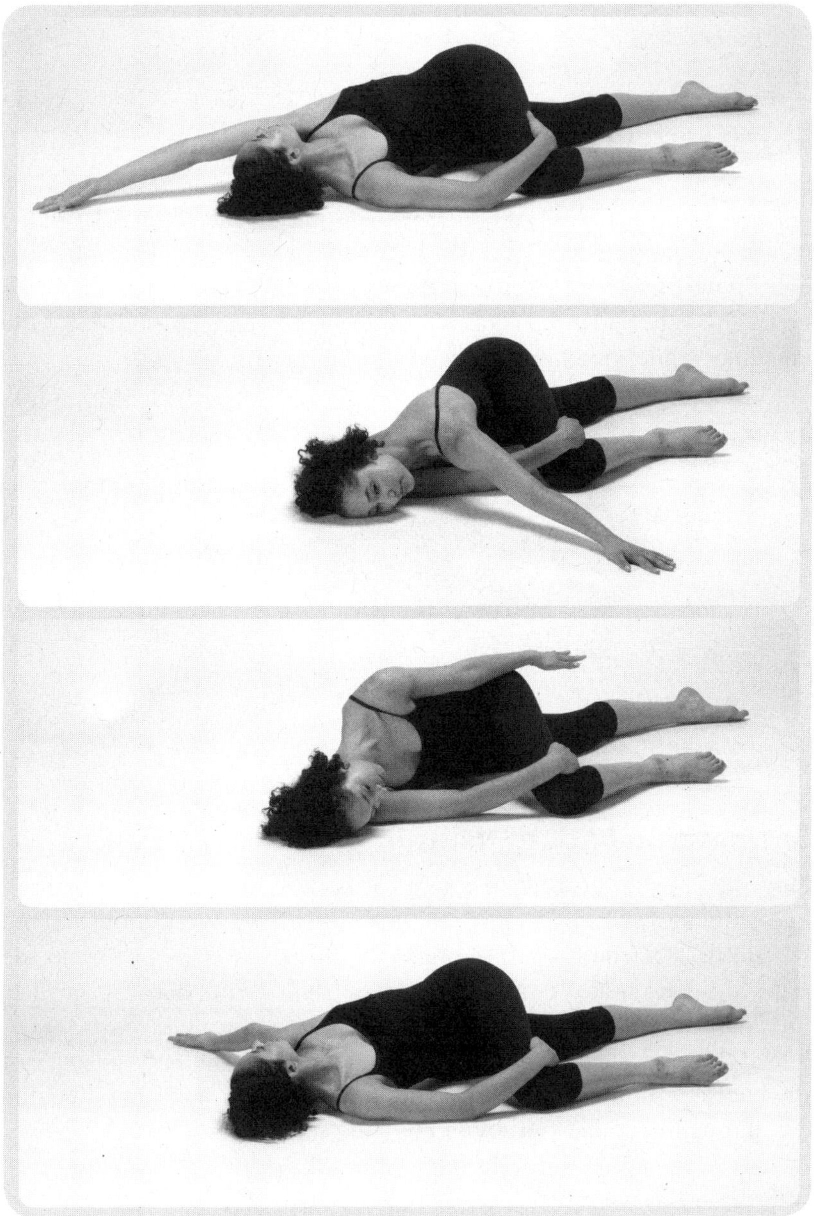

IMAGERY

For *The Clock*, the image of the clock is very useful because it gives spatial orientation to the movement, as well as temporal sequencing. An additional image is that the body is lying in the centre of a series of concentric circles, like a target face in archery. Each circle of the arm should reach to a further circle in the series, with the chest rolling on the bull's eye.

3) The First Spiral Stretch

Finishing in the nine o'clock position, take time to breathe and release tension as the chest and arm soften towards the floor with each exhale. On the inhale, expand the chest and arm with energy and let it go with the exhale. Imagine the outside of the right hip expanding and releasing on each exhale as well.

IMAGERY

For the *Spiral Stretches* (#3 and #4), images of melting, sinking, dropping weight into the floor, and focusing on the breath will all assist with the release of tension and improved range of motion. Imagine the line of energy from the armpit of the extended arm to the hip of the bent leg, elongating, and the spiral of the spine continuing, like a striped barbershop pole.

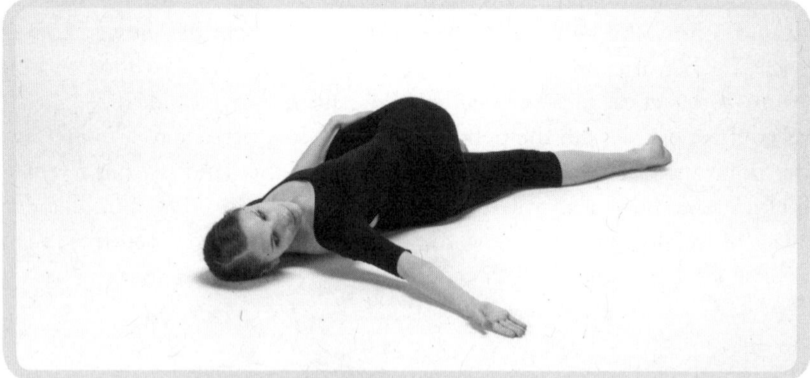

4) The Second Spiral Stretch

There is an important variation of *The First Spiral Stretch* that will be done later in Part Five for the intermediate and advanced levels. Until the dancer has reached that level of work, this variation should be inserted here. Slowly move the arm to a high diagonal, so that it is still close or on the floor, but now the hand is reaching to eleven o'clock. Repeat the breathing while stretching in this new position.

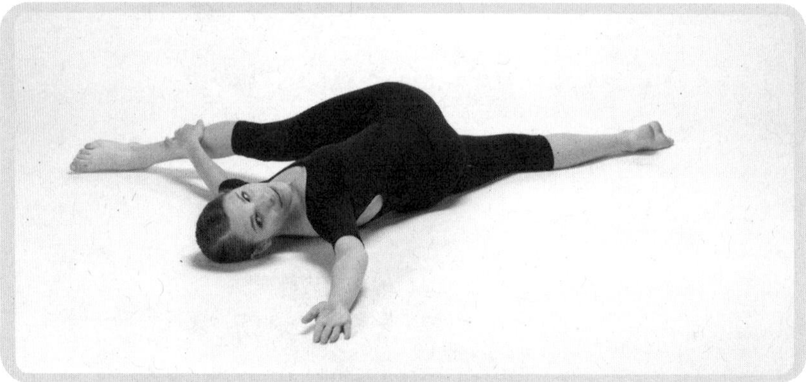

5) Transition Back to Neutral

Fold the left (bottom) leg and bring it underneath the right leg; both knees are now pointing to three o'clock. Initiating from the core, roll the sacrum back to the floor, bringing both knees above the chest and the arms to the floor at the sides of the hips, palms facing down. If needed, use the hands on the floor to realign the spine and head. Take the legs to 90/90 (hip and knee joint both at 90° of flexion), maintain the angle at the knee, keep the pelvis neutral, and return the feet slowly to the floor, continuing to breathe and soften the body surfaces.

Repeat the entire series on the second side.

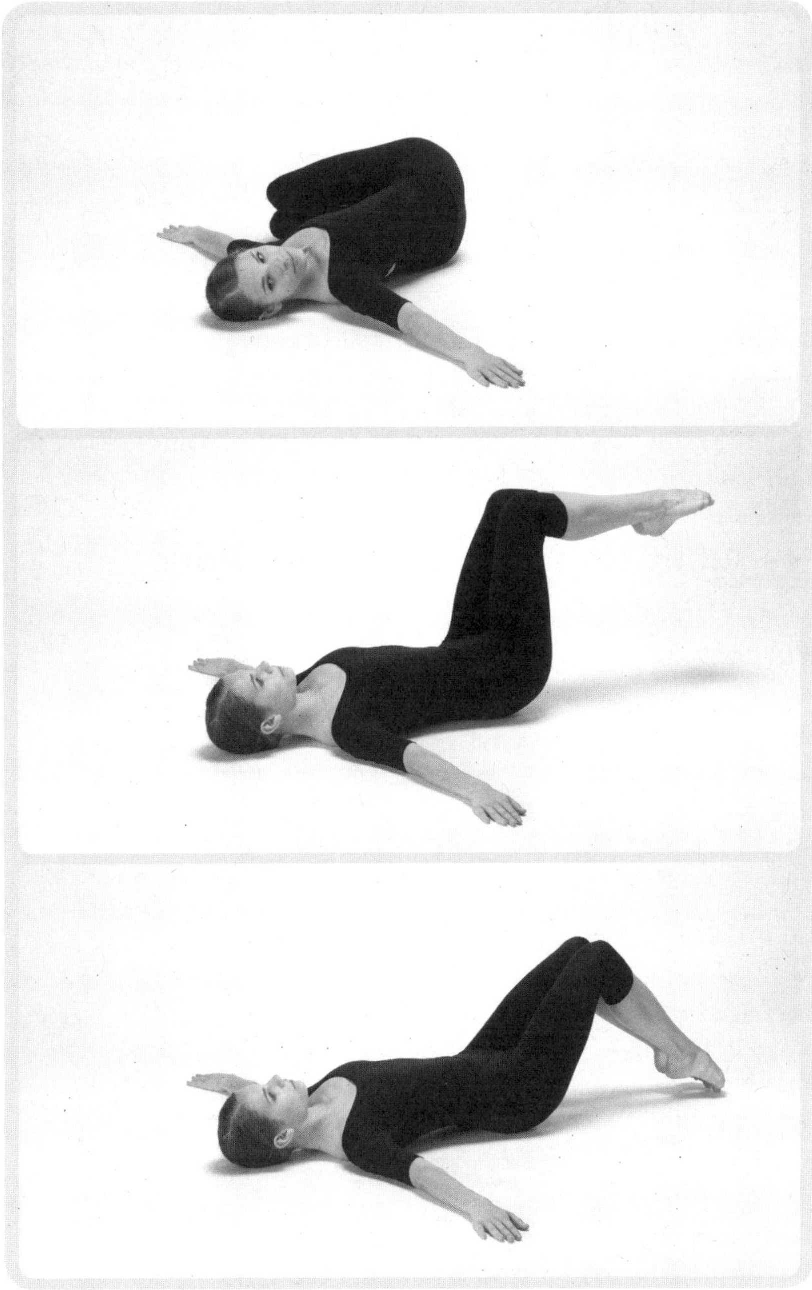

IMAGERY

For *Transition Back to Neutral*, as the sacrum is rolling towards the floor, imagine a large magnet on the sacrum drawing both the sacrum and the navel towards the ground. At the same time, the back of the neck softens and elongates, energy flowing out of the top of the head.

Applications and Transfer to Standing and Travelling Work

If there is excessive tightness and/or incorrect holding patterns in the shoulder joints and shoulder girdles, the alignment of the upper torso is seriously affected. As mentioned above, tightness in the muscles anterior to the shoulder joint will cause rounded shoulders, and in trying to correct this problem, dancers often pull the shoulders back with excessive muscular effort. This causes a chain reaction, resulting in the rib cage being pulled forward on the spine and the muscles between the scapulae going into spasm. There will be detrimental consequences to balance and coordination, as well as aesthetics, as a result.

Notes for Teachers

In *Preparation*, as the thigh moves to the chest, encourage the dancer to bring the knee directly towards the midline of the body (in a proximal direction), rather than allowing the knee to drift out towards the shoulder (in a distal direction). This can assist in recruiting the psoas rather than the more superficial hip flexors, as in *Walking in Space* (Section A, #6, page 5). In the stretches, it is important to make sure the dancer is dropping the shoulder towards the floor, and not just the arm. Essentially, the entire side of the chest should melt towards the floor during the stretches. Dancers who are particularly tight may need to do *The Clock* and the *Spiral Stretches* with both knees fully bent. If dancers experience tingling in the arm during the stretches, adjust the placement of the arm slightly and/or move the head around gently. If the tingling persists, fold the elbow.

H – Additional Foot and Ankle Work

Purpose

The *Ankle Circles* exercise is designed to lubricate all of the joints in the foot and ankle and to prepare them for full motion. The transitions and extensions reinforce awareness of core support (even in isolated foot activity) and space in the joints of the lower limbs. The series also emphasizes the parallel alignment of hip, knee, and foot. The reason that the first set of circles is done with the passive, held leg using a pointed foot, and the second set using a flexed foot, is to give balance to the dorsi and plantar flexors of the ankle. In *Transition Back to Neutral* (#3), the idea of reaching out through the heel, and then pointing the foot by leaving the heel that high and reaching the foot further into the space is to create space in the ankle joint for improved range and function. Finally, the dancer is working on a relaxed sense of the neck and shoulders during leg action.

1) Preparation

Starting from parallel stance, point the right foot so that the big toe touches the floor and the ankle comes into alignment with the tibia (shin bone). Bring the thigh towards the chest, remembering to maintain the sacrum connection to the floor to prevent the pelvis from tucking under. Take hold of the leg by interlocking the fingers of both hands around the shin just under the knee joint. Now take the attention to the left leg and flex the left foot. On the exhale, slide the left leg out along the floor, reaching out the heel and top of the head. Keeping the left foot flexed and the heel in contact with the floor, bend the knee as if doing a parallel demi plié on one foot. In the mind, see the centre of the hip joint, the centre of the knee joint, and the centre of the foot in alignment, with the knee and toes pointing straight up to the ceiling. Now increase the hip flexion, bringing the left leg up to parallel attitude above the hip, with the bottom of the left foot facing the ceiling. Remember to keep the sacrum connected to floor.

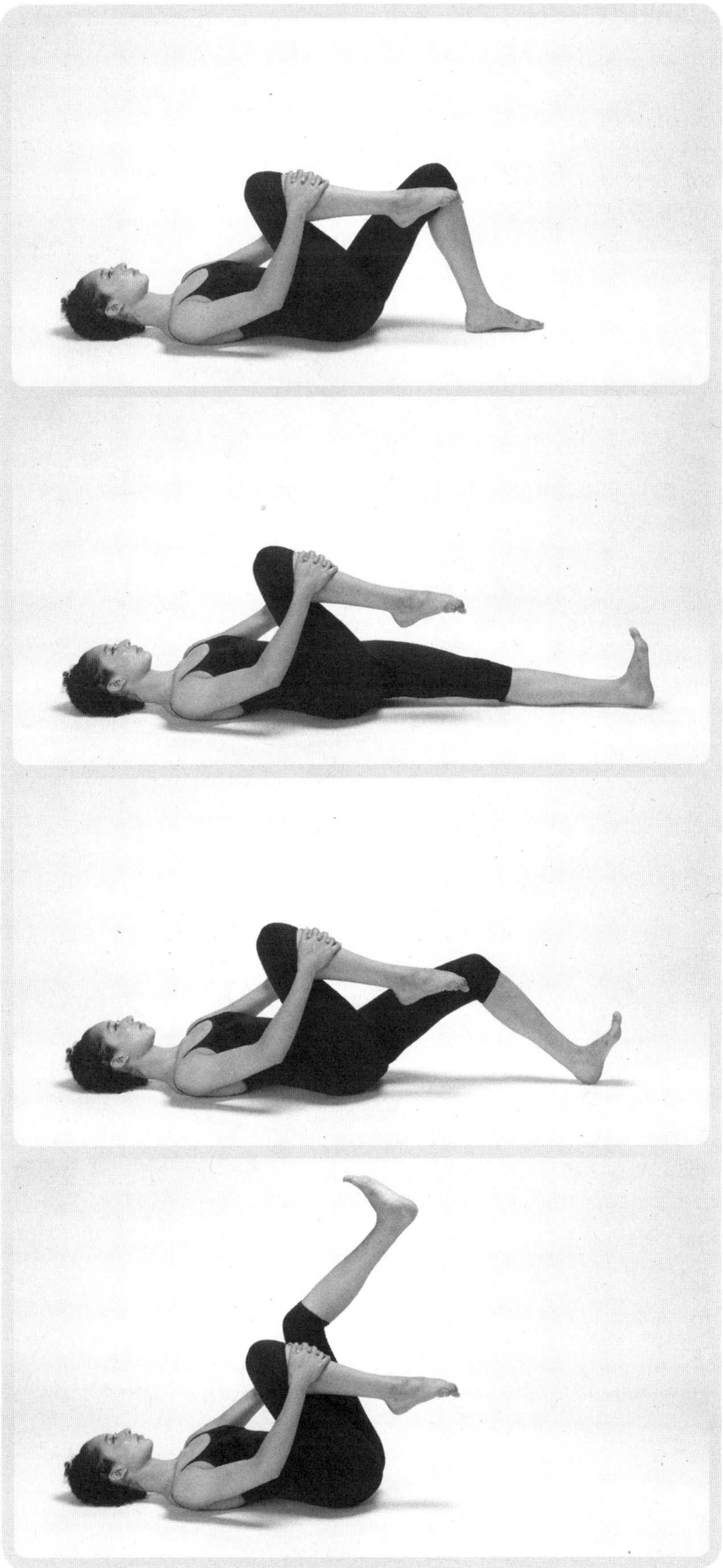

IMAGERY

For *Preparation*, refer to the images in the previous series (*The Clock* preparation). Additionally, as the leg moves to attitude, image a magnet on the back of the sacrum, keeping it attached to the floor to avoid tucking under.

2) Ankle Circles

Using a moderate tempo, circle the left foot outside (counter-clockwise), eight times, making an even, smooth circle, maintaining the parallel alignment of the hip and knee. Think of the size and timing of the circle being symmetrical on both sides. Finish the eighth circle with a flexed foot, and extend the leg as the foot points on counts 1,2; return to the attitude and flex both feet on 3,4. Now do eight circles in the opposite direction (clockwise). Finish once again with a flexed foot, and extend the leg as both feet point.

IMAGERY

During the *Ankle Circles*, imagine oil or grease in the joints of the feet and ankles, and see the bones gliding and sliding. To assist in maintaining the parallel line of both legs, imagine a thin sheet of glass or paper standing vertically along the midline of the body (between the legs if the body is in neutral stance), and keep the inner thighs of both legs touching the glass or paper throughout the ankle circles and transitions. On the extension of the leg after each circling series, imagine air pouring out of the foot on the extension and point, and the sacrum and hip dropping more deeply into the floor, to encourage oppositional energy through the leg.

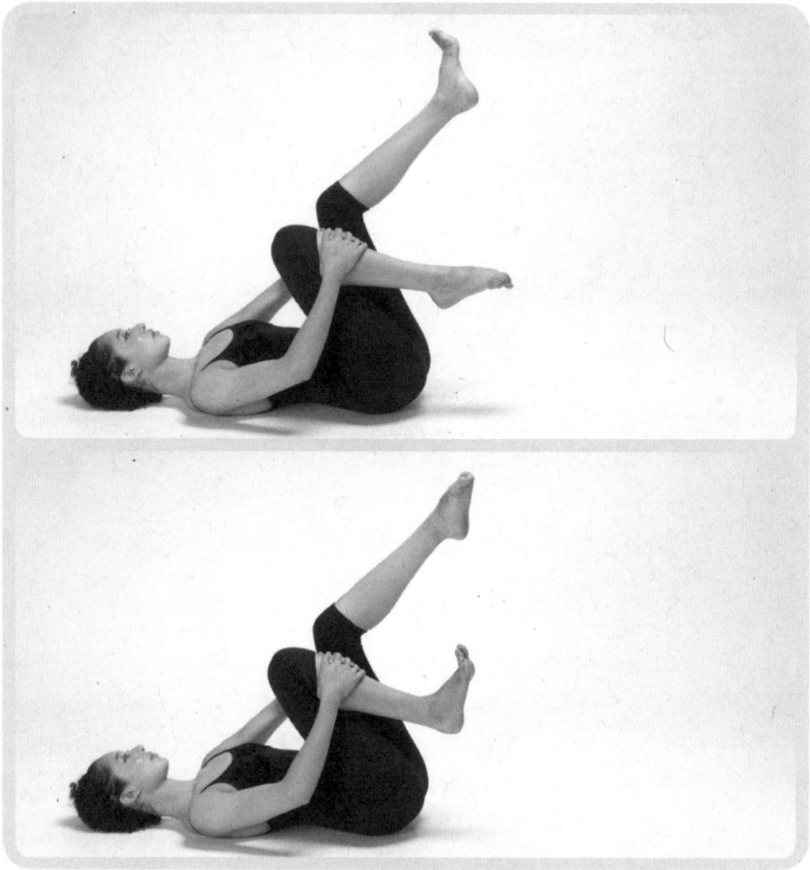

3) Transition Back to Neutral

Flex the left foot, imagining that the heel reaches higher in space towards the ceiling, rather than the toes moving down towards the shin bone. While trying to keep the heel that high in the space, point the foot successionally, reaching the metatarsals and then the toes away from the heel. On the next exhale, slowly lower the parallel leg towards the floor, creating a huge arc with the big toe, narrowing and hollowing, and opening the front of the hip joint (hip flexors releasing). At the same time, energy reaches out the top of the head. As the heel touches the floor, draw the right leg closer to the chest with the hands, feeling the two-way stretch between the legs and separating the inner thighs. Pause for a stretch. Slowly bring the left leg back to neutral stance, then let go of the right leg and return it to neutral stance, maintaining core support throughout.

Repeat the entire series on the second side.

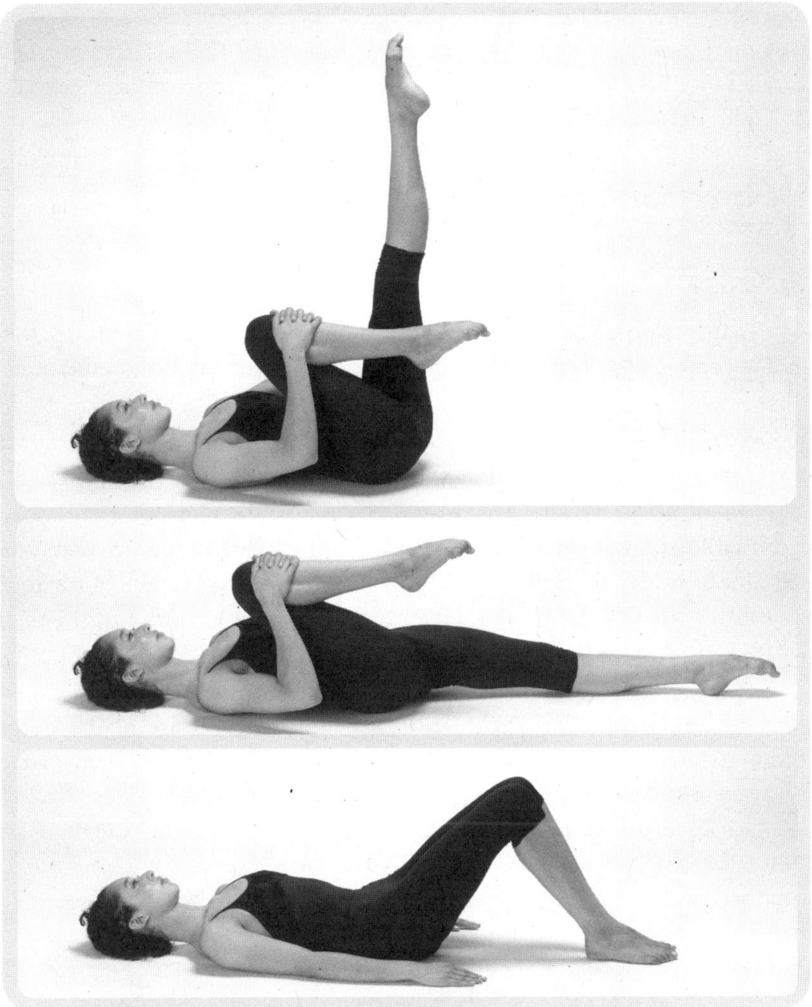

IMAGERY

For *Transition Back to Neutral*, imagine that breath or energy or light is flowing out of the toes and the top of the head in opposite directions, and the waist is narrowing as the leg is lowering towards the floor. The tube of toothpaste image can also be suggested. Imagine that the chest and shoulders are widening as the waist narrows. As the leg is lowering, imagine that the front of the hip joint is taffy and it is elongating and softening as the leg reaches away from the hip socket. During the stretch at the end, imagine that the two legs are like a bow and arrow to encourage the sensation of oppositional stretch.

Applications and Transfer to Standing and Travelling Work

This series is effective in preparing the feet and ankles for standing work prior to weight bearing, which can assist in warming up this area without compression in the joints. It can also pattern good hip/knee/foot alignment for stance.

Notes for Teachers

If the dancer hears or experiences crunching and crackling in the joints, encourage less effort and muscular tension to achieve the circles. This exercise is placed after *U-Shapes for the Ankles* due to the amount of pronation and hypermobility that many dancers have in these joints. This sequencing encourages stability before engaging mobility. Ideally, during this series, the heel of the attitude leg is directly over the sitz bone, but it is better to decrease the height of the attitude (decreased hip flexion) than to allow the pelvis to tuck under. The primary goal is neutral pelvis, and the height of the leg is secondary. Suggest that dancers with knee problems or pain interlock the fingers and hold the leg at the hamstrings, rather than at the shin bone, to minimize any pressure on the knee joint. In the final lowering of the leg to the floor, it will tend to drift laterally rather than directly in line with the hip, due to muscle imbalances. Check at the end that the foot is in direct line with the hip, and that the leg has remained parallel (not turned out) throughout. Also, watch for unnecessary neck and shoulder tension and encourage whole body awareness in isolated tasks.

I – Introducing Turnout

Purpose

The main purpose of this series is to introduce turnout, with neutral pelvis, and appropriate recruitment of the inner and outer thigh musculature.

Peel the Banana is a stretch for the hands and fingers, and is designed to reduce tension patterns in these extremities, due to increased use of the hands and fingers in today's culture (computers, video games, cellphones, remotes).

Legwork in the Diamond is designed to assist in recruiting the deep external rotators of the hip and to stabilize the pelvis while working one leg. The attitudes also encourage a deeper sensory experience of turnout in the hip to bring the heel "forward" in standing work, rather than rotating from the knee to achieve this aesthetic.

Extending the Legs with Turnout is designed to increase recruitment of the inner thigh muscles and hamstrings, and decrease use of the outer thighs (lateral quadriceps) and gluteus maximus. This common imbalance of overuse of outer thighs and underuse of inner thighs in dancers can lead to knee problems such as patellar femoral syndrome. Further, for those dancers with hyperextended knees, this exercise is designed to support working and standing on an extended leg that is not in knee hyperextension by stimulating not only the inner thigh and hamstring activity, but also the connection of the heels.

1) Diamond Stretch

From neutral stance, relax the legs open so that the bottoms of the feet are together and the legs form an open diamond. Focusing on the breathing, allow the weight of the legs to drop open, while maintaining neutral spine.

IMAGERY

For *Diamond Stretch*, imagine the legs are very heavy, so that gravity is assisting the stretch.

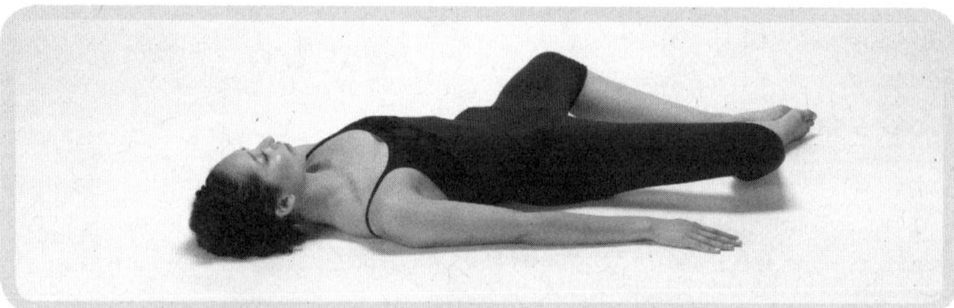

2) Peel the Banana

Folding the right elbow, bring the right hand up to the front of the right shoulder with the palm facing the body. With the left hand, take hold of the fingers of the right hand, with the insides of the palms facing each other. As if peeling a banana, begin to unfold the fingers, the wrist, and the forearm, arriving at an extended arm, palm facing the ceiling, hand above the shoulder. Maintaining the stretch, reach the thumb out to the side.

The right shoulder should stay wide and dropped on the floor. After a thirty-second stretch, shake the hand out and repeat on the left side. Finish with both arms at the sides near the hips, palms facing down.

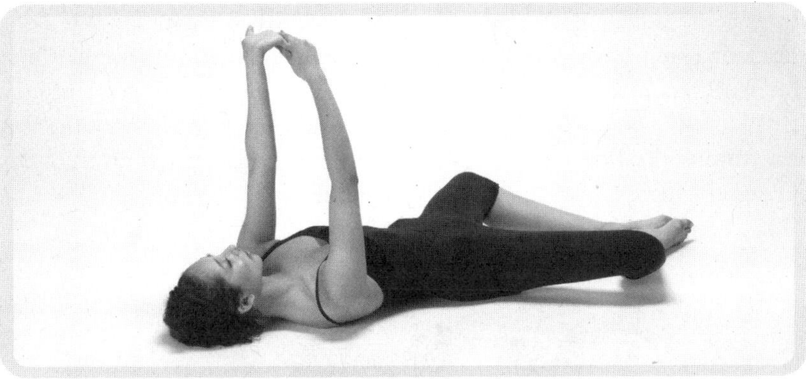

IMAGERY

For *Peel the Banana*, imagine the hand and fingers becoming long and wide so that by the end of the stretch the hand is a catcher's mitt.

3) Legwork in the Diamond

Bring the legs to grand plié position; that is, flex both ankles fully, heels touching and just off the floor, fifth toe and distal metatarsal head on the floor. (A) Points and flexes: Point the feet on counts 1,2, keeping the heels just off the floor and opening the inner thighs so that the little toes stay in place on the floor; then flex the feet on 3,4, bringing the heels back together, maintaining the width of the inner thighs. Do eight repetitions, ending in the pointed position. (B) Small attitude lifts: From the pointed, open position, do alternating lifts of the foot off the floor, lifting the foot on count 1, and lowering on 2. The movement should initiate as a rotary action in the hip socket so that the thigh does not lift higher in the space, but the foot comes just off the floor as the femur rotates, maintaining the flexion angle at the knee. The foot will only lift a small amount if done correctly. Do eight repetitions in total.

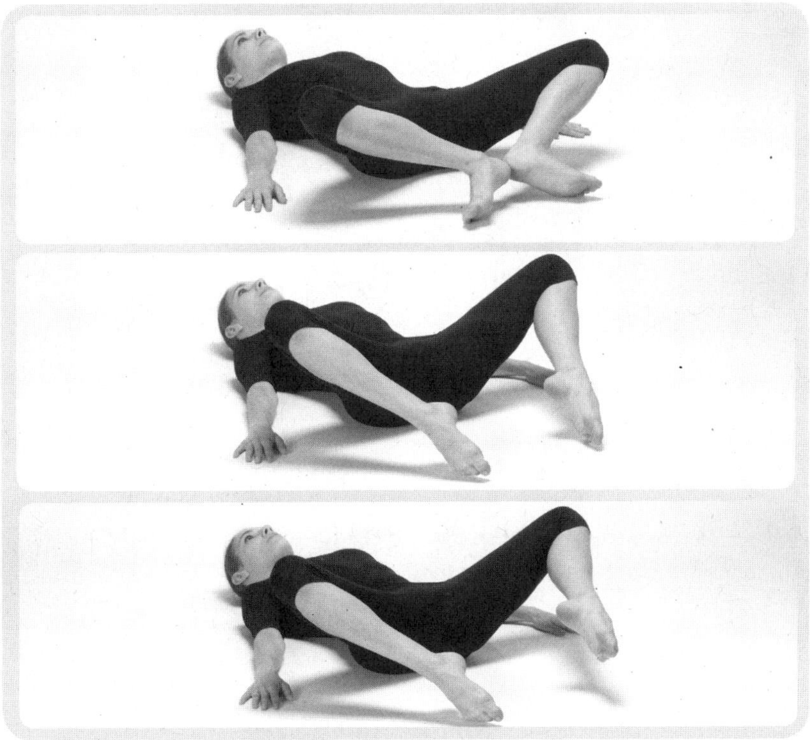

IMAGERY

For *Legwork in the Diamond* – Points and flexes, imagine the thighs getting wider with each point and staying that wide with each flex, so that the space between the femurs continues to expand. Also, imagine that the heels reach away from the pelvis, not up towards the ceiling, with each flex.

For *Legwork in the Diamond* – Small attitude lifts, the action of the leg is similar to the arm if one was pulling a cork out of a bottle, creating a rotary movement at the hip joint, not a lift of the entire leg away from the floor. Also, imagine that the standing hip becomes heavier and cannot tip off the floor.

4) Extending the Legs with Turnout

Keeping the feet pointed (from the end of #3B), bring the big toes together, maintaining the open diamond in the thighs. As if someone were holding the feet and pulling them out away from the body, elongate the legs along the floor, reaching out with the feet, and gathering the inner thighs. Once the heels touch, keep them connected and continue the process until the legs are fully extended and turned out, with the feet pointed. Flex the feet, maintaining the heel connection, and send the heels away from the body. Rotate the legs parallel and return to neutral stance.

IMAGERY

For *Extending the Legs with Turnout*, imagine large magnets on the inner thighs drawing together during the movement, while soft silk or hot water is running down the outer thighs. Imagine that a person is holding the feet and pulling/dragging the legs into the extended position, as if the movement were occurring without conscious effort or control. Imagine the buttocks like unbaked dough, softening onto the floor. At the point when the heels touch, pause and imagine squirting crazy glue between the heels, to keep them connected throughout the extension. One can also imagine that the person holding the feet is actively pressing the heels together. Finally, imagine the toothpaste tube, so that energy is shooting out of the head as the legs are extending and the waist is narrowing.

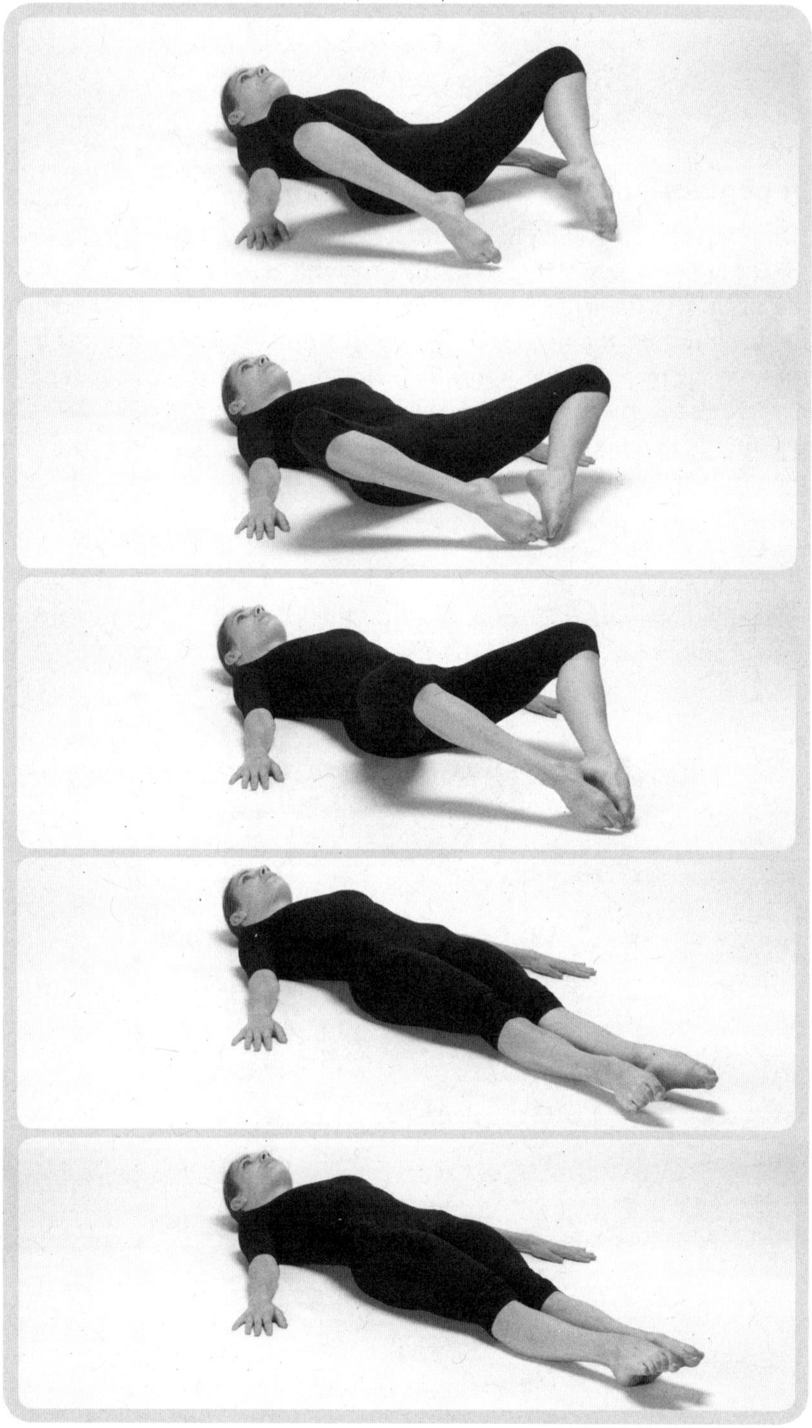

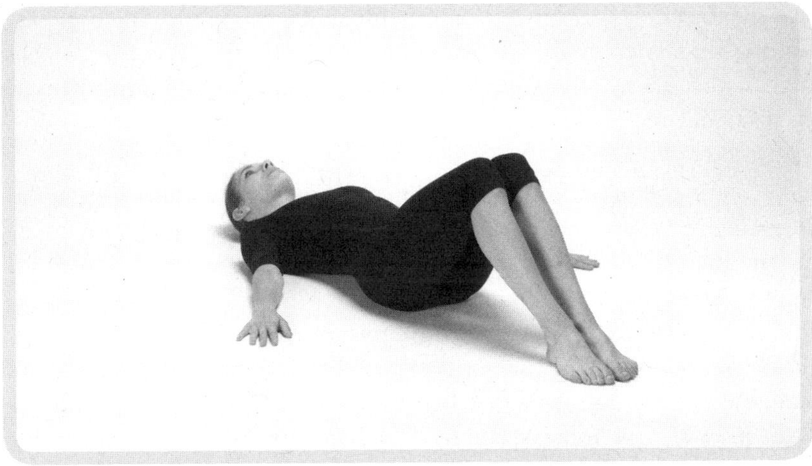

Applications and Transfer to Standing and Travelling Work

Peel the Banana is important for expressivity in dance. If the hands are tense or gripped, all of the arm movements will lose their fluidity and lines of energy, blocking expression and artistry. Hand tension can also inhibit movements that require weight-bearing on the arms and partnering work. Dancers' hands need to be as mobile and articulate as their feet.

Legwork in the Diamond informs the dancer about rotation from deep inside the hip socket, and not from peripheral indicators such as the angle of the feet. It also gives the dancer a sensory cue for finding turnout in the gesture leg with a stable pelvis when working on one leg.

The images used in *Extending the Legs with Turnout* can be directly applied to standing work. In stance, the imaginary person is now holding the waist and lifting the pelvis away from the heels as the inner thighs are drawn together by magnets. As with lying, the focus is not on straightening the knees, but in elongating the legs and increasing the distance between feet and pelvis. The heels remain glued together and the silk or hot water continues pouring down the outer legs to inhibit hyperextending or jamming the knees. At the top of the movement, the pelvic floor should have a light pouring down directly over the heels.

Notes for Teachers

In *Peel the Banana*, make sure that dancers do not force the elbow into extension. Dancers with hyperextended elbows, should do this hand stretch with slight elbow flexion. Dancers with hypermobility in the fingers, should avoid this stretch altogether. Instead, they can do isometric strength work by placing the hands in prayer position in front of the chest and pressing the fingers together.

For the remaining exercises in this series, if dancers are having difficulty stabilizing the pelvis, have them place the hands around the waist (as they did for *Undercurves*), and they will be able to sense when the pelvis is rocking. When dancers are in the grand plié, check that the ankle is fully dorsiflexed, and it is not only the metatarsals that are creating the foot position. Further, the heels must not be pressed as high as possible, which causes torque at the knee and can contribute to foot pronation. Check that the foot is in alignment with the shin. If dancers are having difficulty finding the inner thigh activity while *Extending the Legs with Turnout*, suggest that they actively press the heels together at the point of heel contact, and maintain this pressure for the remainder of the extension. Continue to encourage the softening of the outer surface muscles.

It can be useful to do some standing visualization work to accompany *Extending the Legs with Turnout*. The dancers can be given the following instructions: Come to standing in first position, turned out. Take some time to experience the alignment of the pelvis and the organization of the legs in relation to the spine. Move into a demi plié, imagining a huge diamond widening the knees out over the feet. Without thinking about straightening the legs, imagine that the pelvis is floating upward as the waist narrows and hollows, and that the magnets on the inner thighs are being drawn together and forward. Imagine the thighs sliding down the front of the leg and the buttocks sliding down the back of the leg as the inner thighs gather under the rising pelvic floor.

PART TWO LEGWORK AND CORE SUPPORT

2

Opening Remarks

This section has three central goals. The first goal is to encourage use of the deep external rotators for turnout. Work for developing turnout is introduced lying supine with the hip joint in flexion to reduce gluteus maximus contribution and to emphasize the use of the deep rotators (piriformis, gemellus superior, gemellus inferior, obturator internus, obturator externus, and quadratus femoris). Because the gluteus maximus is a hip extensor, it is less likely to contribute to external rotation when the hip is in flexion, thereby encouraging the deep rotators to engage. The second goal is to develop appropriate lower leg alignment for standing and travelling work. In these exercises, the foot and knee are patterned to function in a corridor in order to develop this organization on both a muscular and neuromuscular level. When the knee is flexed, the ligaments will allow for additional rotation at the knee, causing the feet to be behind the knees in standing demi plié. This exercise is designed to pattern hip external rotation in stance, so that the weight-bearing joints (hip, knee, foot) have skeletal support. Additionally, this series provides visual feedback about this alignment. The third goal of this series is to organize the core with the legs, and to integrate core support into the use of hip rotation.

A – Integrating Standing and Gesture Legs with the Core

Purpose

The primary purpose of this entire sequence is to teach efficient use of the external rotators for turnout, and to emphasize leg alignment and core support in relation to turnout. The focus of this section is to help the dancer understand that rotation is an action, not a position, and that it requires ongoing activity. The series begins at 45° so that there is no excessive stress on the hamstrings, and it is therefore easier to maintain neutral pelvis. The flexing and pointing of the feet adds additional work for the feet and ankles, as well as providing variety. It also gives the dancer information about the alignment of the foot, knee, and hip in two configurations. By the time the dancer is ready for the 90° variations, the challenges of maintaining neutral pelvis, core support, and lower leg alignment increase.

Lowering and Raising the Leg on various counts is designed to teach the action of grand battement with the pelvis stabilized for standing work. The action of stabilizing the pelvis in conjunction with large gestures and direct spatial intention is critical to much of the large range-of-motion legwork learned in dance. While gravity acts differently on the leg once the body is in stance, it is still valuable to provide the experience of isolated hip action (flexion/extension) for the grand battement. The stretching at the end of this section is intended to allow recuperation time for the leg muscles, and to address flexibility when these muscles are warm.

The use of the breath and, in particular, the vocalization during the abdominal sequences, is to ensure that the breath is (1) not held, which will contribute to bracing with the superficial abdominal muscles, and (2) involving the diaphragm, and not only occurring in the upper chest. While use of breath is important in all of the C-I Training work, it is particularly crucial for all of the exercises designed to encourage recruitment of core support and abdominal muscles.

The Plié Reach Series fully integrates core support, leg movement corresponding to plié, and external hip rotation into one action. The isometric engagement of the abdominals, coupled with the various leg actions, teaches pelvic stabilization while the legs are in motion. Both this exercise and the earlier rotations in attitude (*Rotating In and Out*, Variations 1 and 2) emphasize the foot/knee/hip relationship to prevent injuries to the knees and ankles caused by misalignment.

Note: This entire sequence is done on the right side, and then repeated on the left side. It is not as long as it looks!

1) Rotating In and Out

From neutral stance, flex the right foot and, on the exhale, slide the leg out along the floor. Maintaining neutral pelvis, keep that leg straight and flex the hip to approximately 45°, so that the knees are at the same level and the insides of the knees are touching. In this position, point the foot on 1, rotate the hip fully out on 2, flex the foot on 3, and rotate the hip in (beyond parallel) on 4, exploring the full range of movement of hip joint rotation. Do four repetitions.

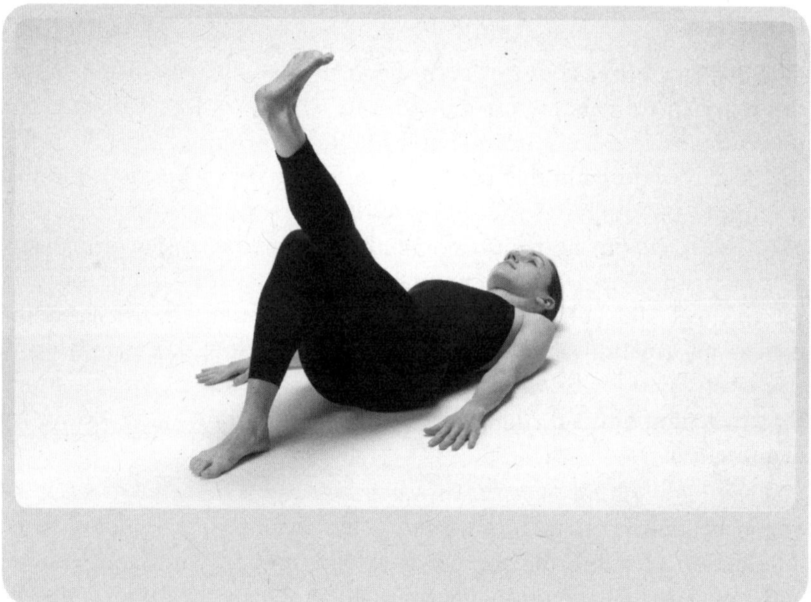

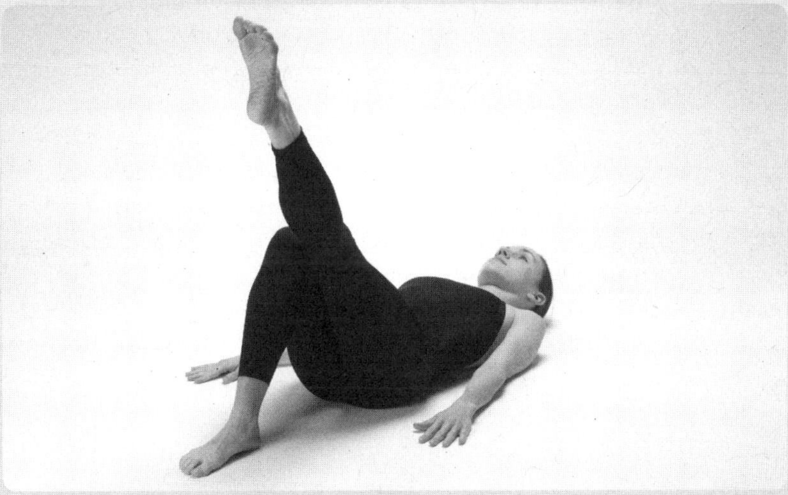

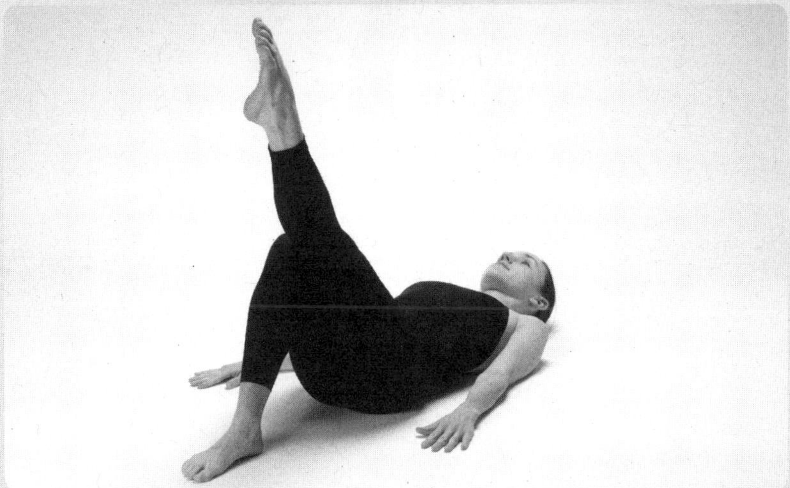

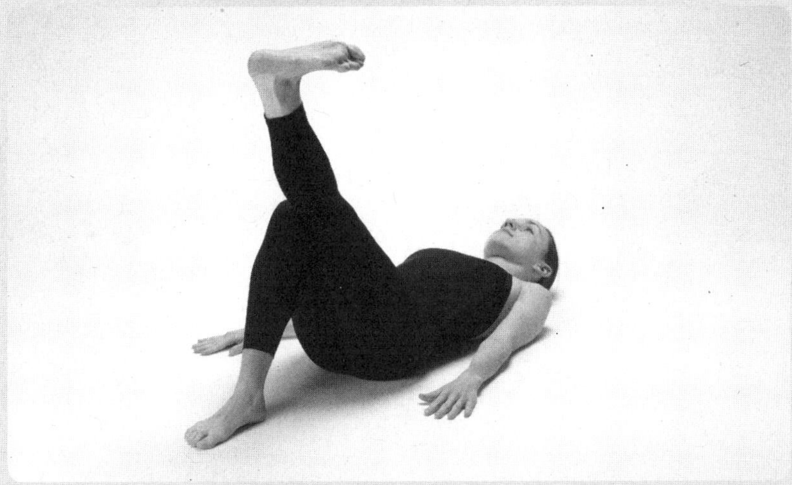

IMAGERY

At the beginning of *Rotating In and Out*, as the leg slides out along the floor, imagine energy or light pouring out of the heel and the top of the head simultaneously. During the rotation series, imagine the crease at the hip of the standing leg sinking and deepening. Imagine the knee of that leg attached to the ceiling by a string, so that it does not drop open into external rotation. The head continues to actively reach along the floor, as the waist narrows and hollows, and the shoulders widen as they do in count 2 of the *Arm Series on 8*. With each flex and point, see the heel elongating further away from the hip socket. Imagine the ball and socket as oily or slick, and then see the action of the femoral head as a rolling, continuous movement in the socket—a greasy ball rolling in a bowl.

Attitude Variation 1 (on 4 counts) – Transition: From the final turned-in position, come to parallel with the gesture leg on 1, bend the knee 2, and float the leg to parallel front attitude with the foot above the hip joint 3,4, while maintaining neutral pelvis. Repeat the sequence above in the attitude. It is important to focus the effort on the rotary action at the hip joint, so that the foot remains in line with the knee throughout the series. On count 4, the hip should come to parallel only (not beyond) so that the dancer has visual feedback about the knee/foot relationship. Do four repetitions. Transition: Keep the foot flexed and extend the leg towards the ceiling 1, 2, rotate out from the hip 3, 4.

IMAGERY

For the attitude variations, imagine that the knee and foot of the attitude leg are caught in a narrow corridor so that the lower leg/knee cannot rotate, and the rotary aspect is isolated in the hip joint.

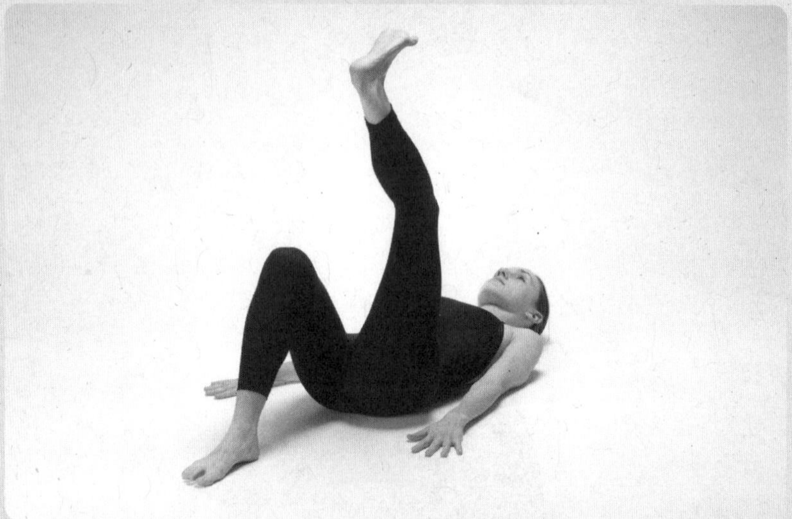

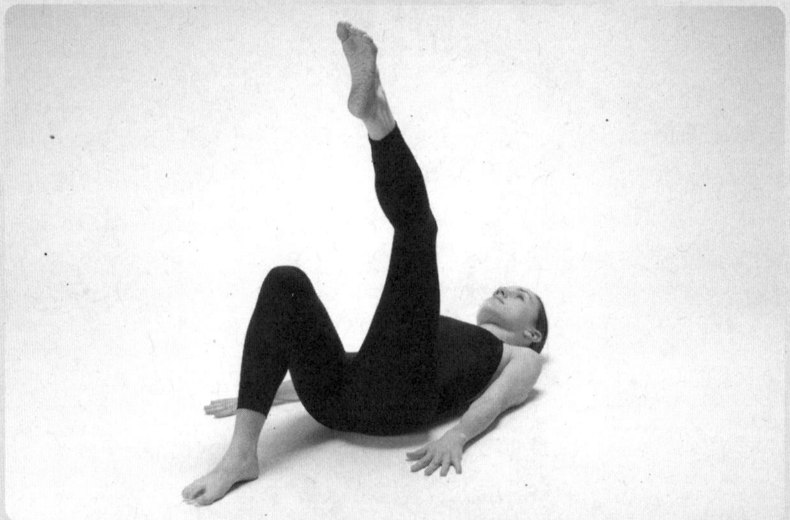

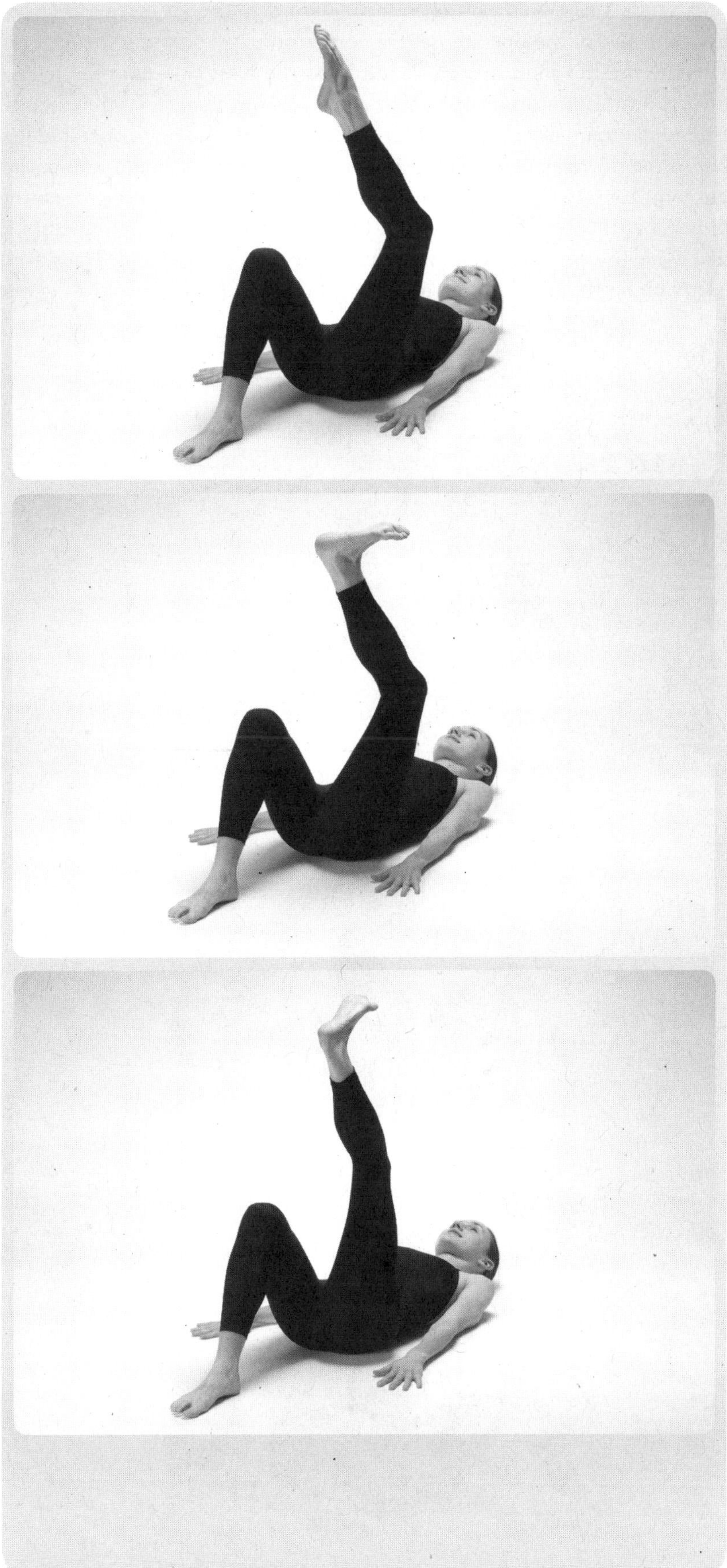

Attitude Variation 2 (on 6 counts) – For a more advanced variation, from the end of the opening sequence, transition by pointing the foot on 1, rotate the hip joint out on 2, and bend the knee and float the leg to turned out front attitude with foot above the hip joint 3,4, while maintaining neutral pelvis. Flex the foot on 1, rotate parallel on 2, open the leg out to the side, staying parallel 3,4, rotate the hip joint out and adduct the hip joint back to the turned out front attitude 5,6. Repeat this six-count phrase, but this time, point the foot on count 1; do two more repetitions, first with the foot flexed and second with the foot pointed. Transition: Maintaining the hip external rotation, extend the leg towards the ceiling 1,2, flex the foot 3,4.

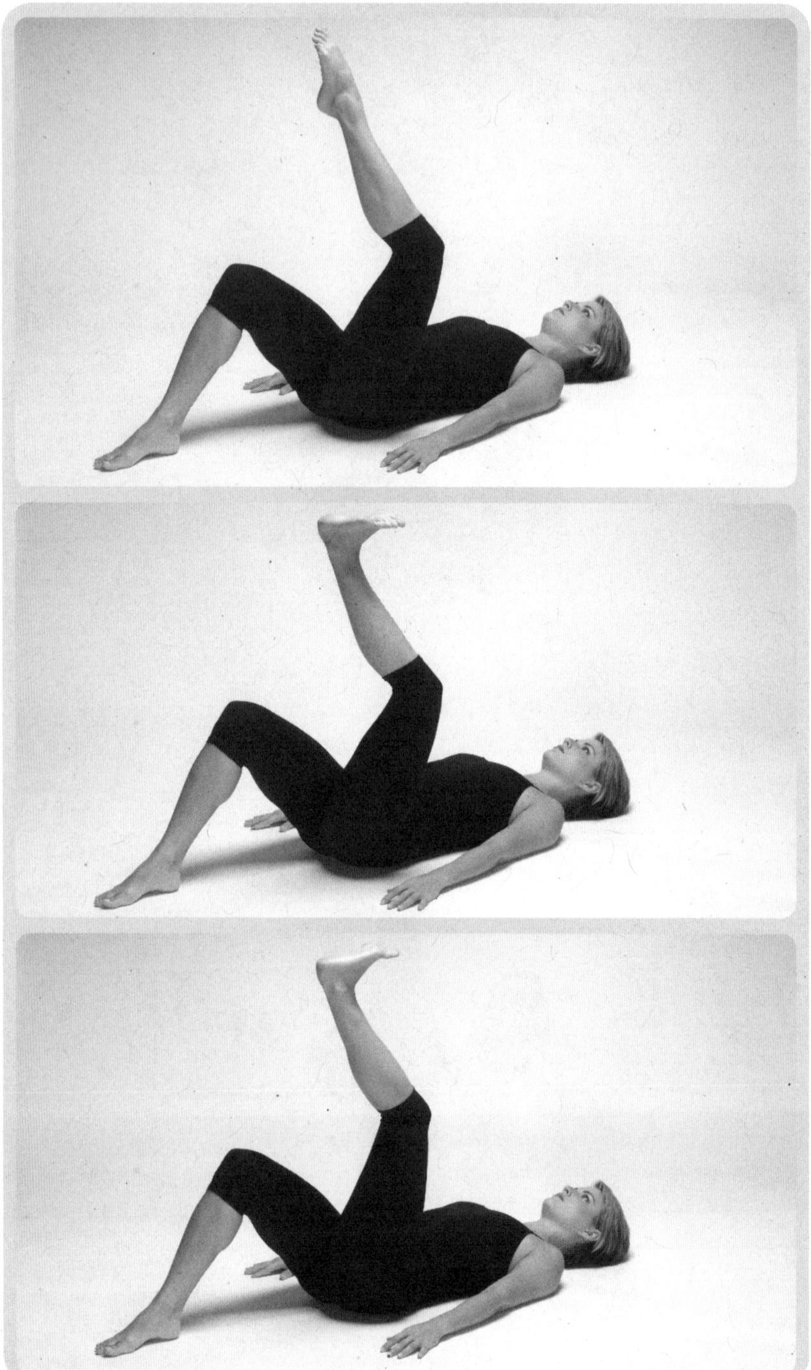

IMAGERY

The *Attitude Variation 2 (on 6 counts)* presents greater challenges to the stabilization of the standing leg, and so the images provided previously are increasingly important. Additionally, as the gesture leg opens side on 3,4, imagine the sacrum on the standing side becoming heavier. At the moment that the gesture leg turns out on count 5, imagine that the action of external rotation initiates the return of the leg back to the front attitude, so that the action of hip adduction is paired with external rotation.

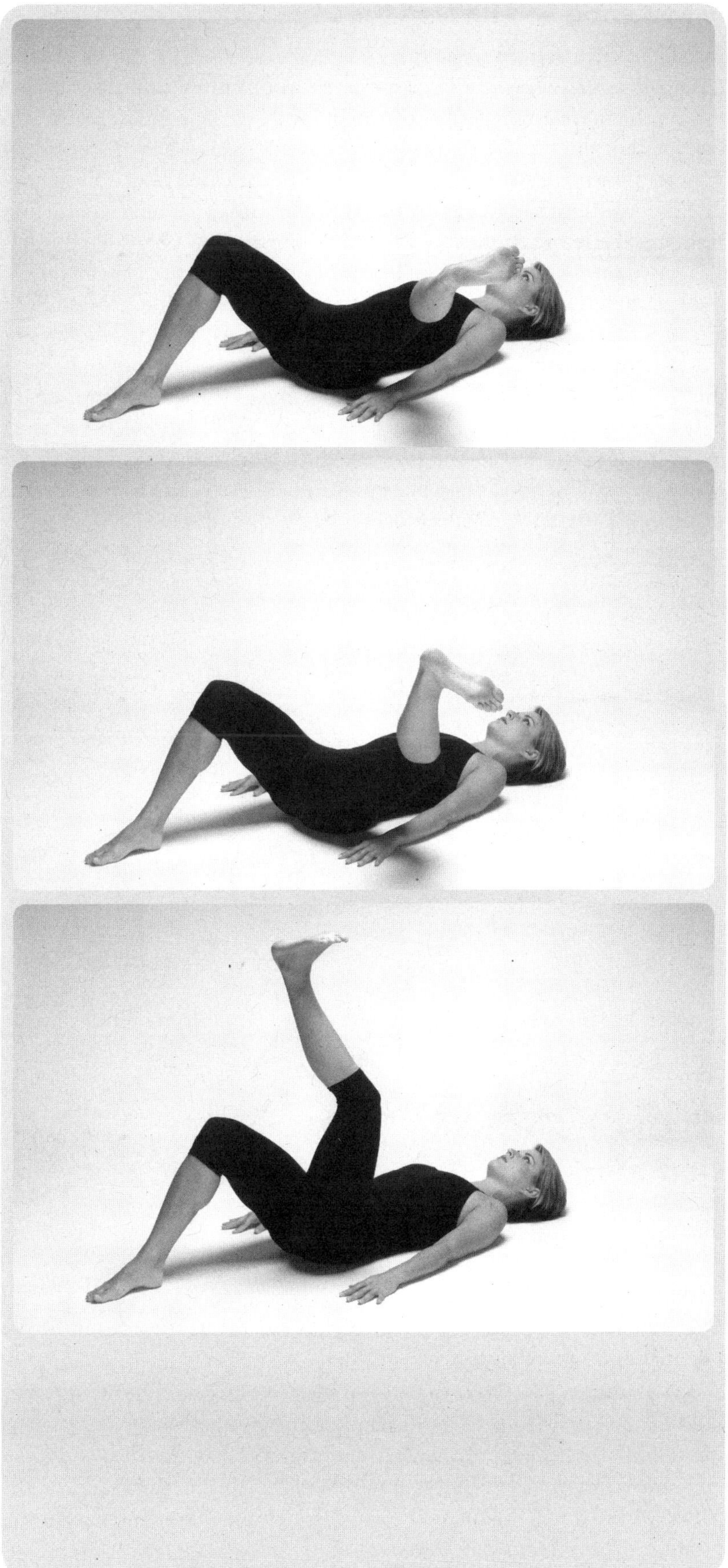

2) Lowering and Raising the Leg

From the final transition at the end of Variation 1 or 2: (A) On the exhale, lower the leg in a large arc away from the torso until it arrives just off the floor, ensuring that the inner thighs make contact (so that the leg does not drift to the side as it is lowering) 1,2,3, point the foot on 4. This motion replicates lowering the leg back to stance from a développé devant or grand battement devant. On the inhale, reverse the action, bringing the leg back up towards the ceiling, turned out and elongated 1,2,3, flex on 4. Once again, the inner thighs should make contact during the movement, and the sacrum should remain on the floor throughout. Do four repetitions. (B) Continue the action of (A), lowering and raising the leg on two counts for each action, rather than four counts, keeping the foot pointed. This increase in tempo makes the stabilization of the pelvis and spine more challenging. (C) For a more advanced variation, lower the leg on three counts and raise the leg on one count, keeping the foot pointed. This dynamic replicates the energy of grand battement, and further challenges the stabilization of the pelvis and spine.

IMAGERY

For *Lowering and Raising the Leg*, imagine a thin sheet of glass standing vertically along the inside edge of the standing leg. During the series, imagine the standing leg actively pressing against this glass. The gesture leg must stay in contact with this sheet of glass throughout each lowering and each lift. Imagine an increase of the narrowing and hollowing as the leg lowers, and an increase of the weight of the sacrum as the leg lifts. As the leg lowers, one can also imagine taffy in the front of the hip joint, softening and elongating, to prevent excess tension. Energy or light should continue shooting out of the foot. As the timing shifts and the leg lift is done at a much faster tempo, these images are increasingly important for stabilizing the pelvis.

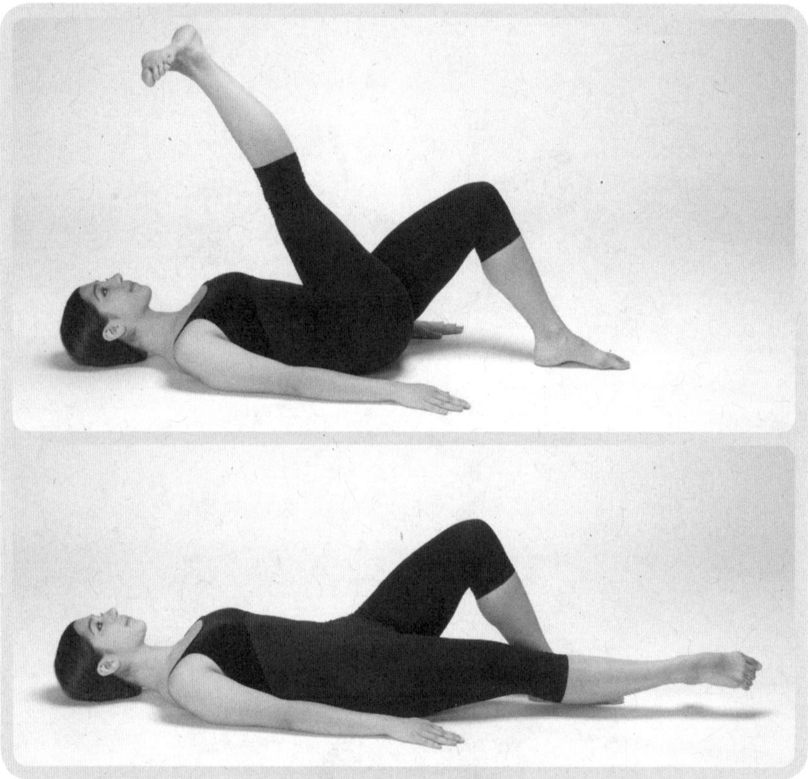

3) Flexibility Series

One can choose to do any or all of the following stretches; it is not essential to do them all to receive benefit.

(A) Hamstrings – From the end of lowering and raising the leg, take hold of the right leg with both hands, either at the calf or the back of the thigh, bring the leg to parallel, and slightly relax the foot and knee. Slide the standing (left) leg out along the floor (this helps to stabilize the pelvis on the floor). Maintain a passive stretch for the hamstrings in this position for approximately thirty seconds.

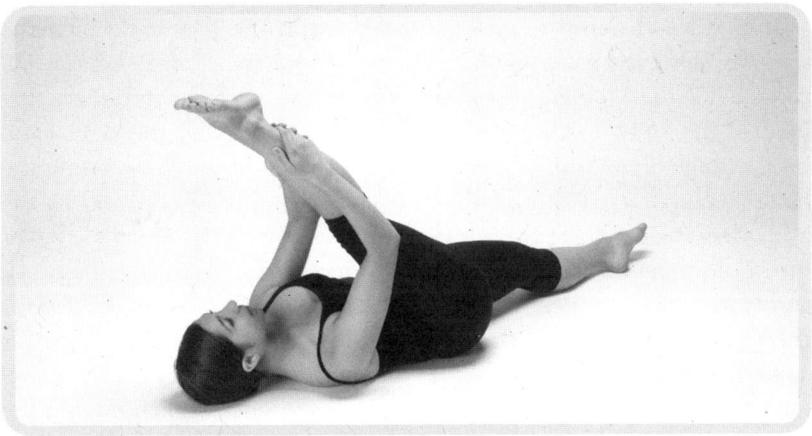

(B) Hamstrings with Leg Across – Open the leg out slightly to the right, and draw it a little higher, increasing the hip flexion. Maintaining this height, slowly draw the leg back across the body towards the opposite (left) shoulder, emphasizing the stretch of the lateral hamstrings. Maintain a passive stretch in this position for approximately thirty seconds.

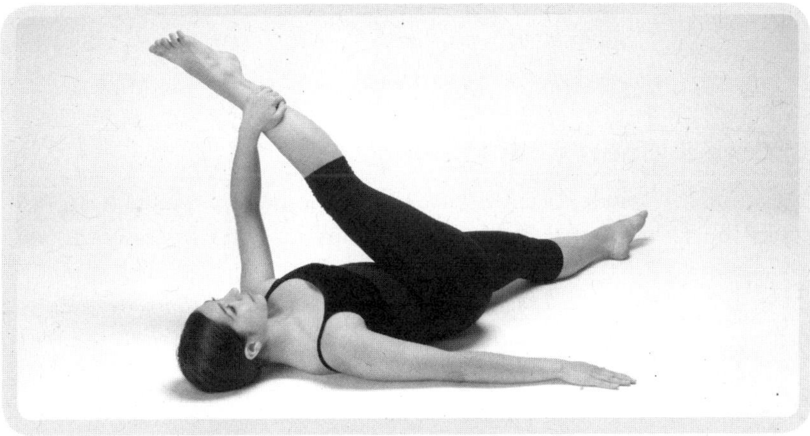

(C) Over-Crossed Passé – Bring the standing (left) leg back to neutral parallel stance. Bend the gesture (right) leg, turn it out fully, and fold it across the standing leg in what can be called "over-crossed passé," so that the outer shin is resting on the left thigh. Then bring the legs towards the chest and hold onto the left leg under the hamstrings, targeting the piriformis for a thirty-second stretch.

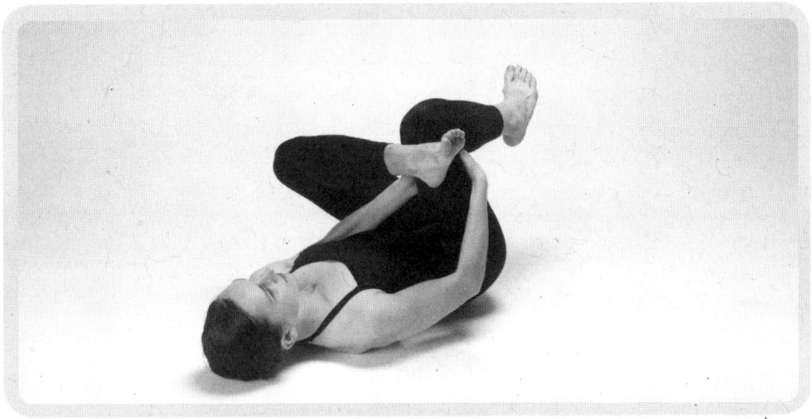

IMAGERY

For *Flexibility Series*, image the breath flowing into the areas of tension or tightness on the inhale, and then see the tension leaving the body on the exhale. Imagine the weight of the limb being stretched sinking into the stretch, not being pulled with force.

(D) Attitude Across – Release the hold on the leg, and return the standing (left) leg back on the floor in neutral stance, maintaining the passé. Bring the right leg up towards the chest into a front attitude, taking hold of the right ankle with the left hand, and placing the right hand on the thigh. Slide the standing (left) leg out along the floor. Using the hands to encourage the turnout, slowly move the attitude across the body, drawing the right knee in front of the left shoulder. Keep the pelvis on the floor, especially the right hip. It is important to stabilize the pelvis and to remain externally rotated, or the stretch will not be effective for the target muscles (gluteus medius and minimus). Hold the stretch for approximately thirty seconds. From the end of the final stretch of choice, return the left leg to neutral stance, arms at the sides of the body on the floor, and extend the right leg towards the ceiling, turned out.

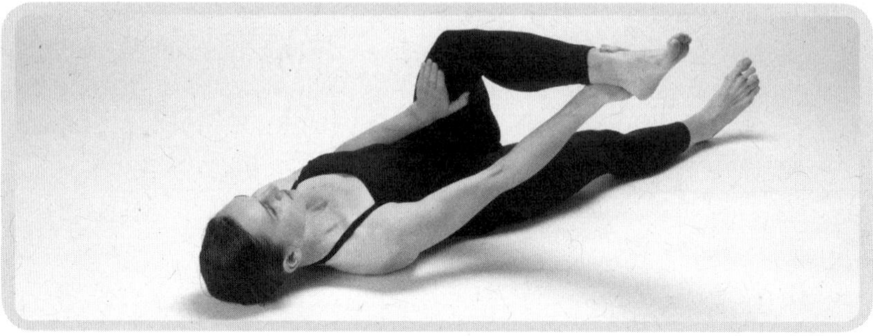

4) Core Support with Moving Legs

Variation 1 – Touch Reach Series: Lower the gesture (right) leg to 45°, rotate the hip to parallel, and connect the insides of the knees. Narrowing and hollowing to initiate the movement, curl the head and shoulders entirely off the floor. Ideally, the top of the head points towards the ceiling, and there is a space the size of a small apple between the chin and chest. Lift the arms so that they are in a rounded oval parallel to the floor, hands behind the hamstrings. Extend the left leg out to 45° to match the right leg. Do NOT stop in this position—immediately begin the touch/reach movement. On count 1, inhale and bend both knees, keeping the thighs at 45°, touching the toes to the floor. On count 2, extend both knees so that the legs reach back to the starting position; exhale on this action, increasing the narrowing and hollowing, and vocalize a long, deep, low-sounding "Huh." Do eight to sixteen repetitions. At the end, bend both knees and return to neutral stance in the legs, torso, and arms.

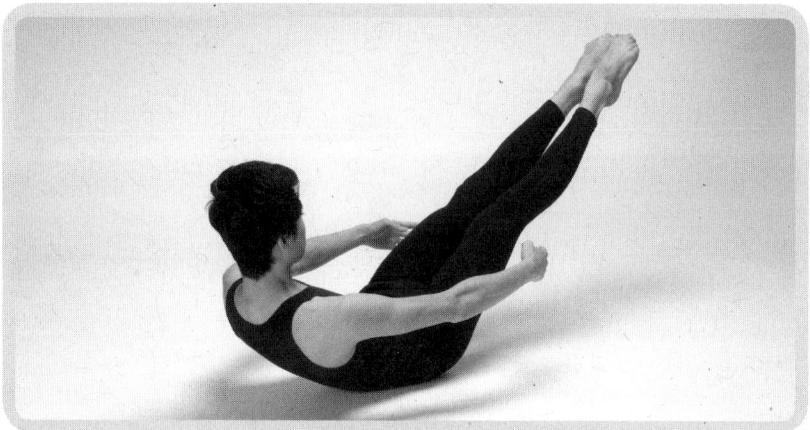

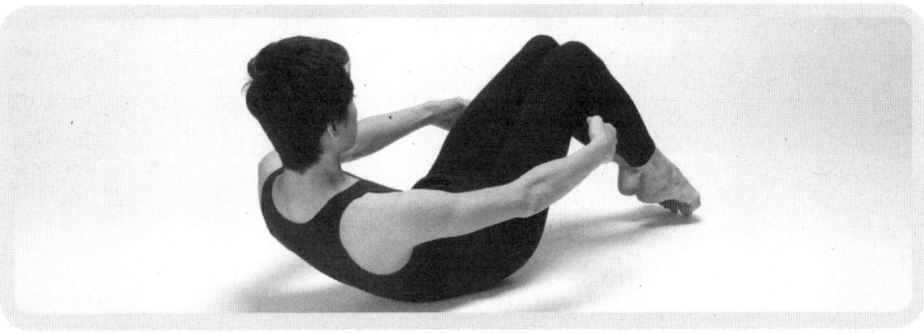

For an advanced variation that involves the obliques, begin in the starting position of Touch Reach Series. The feet draw a tear drop and circle underneath on the bending of the knees, so that on the extension on count 2, one leg is turned in, one leg is turned out. To increase difficulty, the body can rotate in the direction of the top leg, so that it is in opposition to the twist in the pelvis.

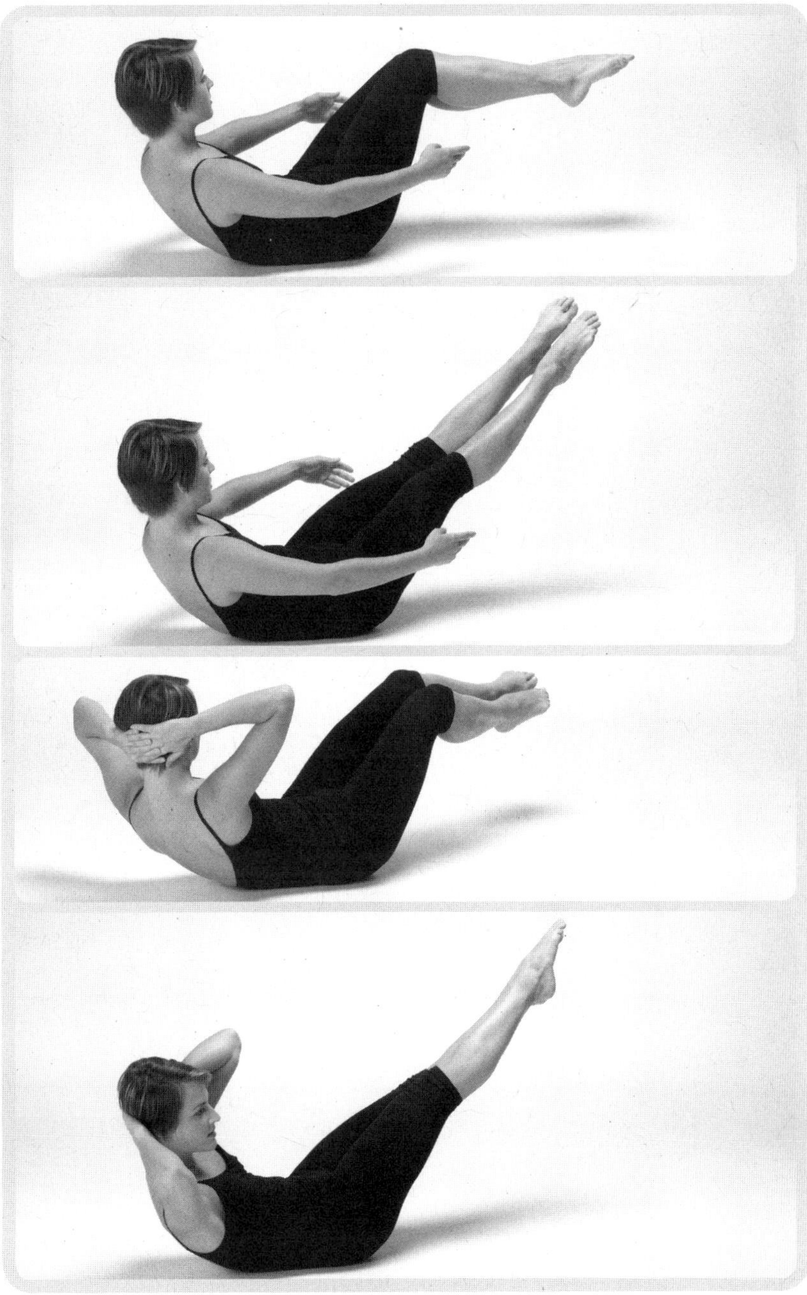

IMAGERY

For *Core Support with Moving Legs*, the toothpaste tube is a great image for all of the abdominal exercises. The waist continues to hollow and narrow on the exhale, and the head continues its reach up and out towards the ceiling. It is also useful to imagine the giant ice cream scoop scooping out the lower abdominals with each leg reach. Imagine that the lumbar spine and sacrum are glued to the floor the entire time, and that the upper back is floating up off the floor. Shoulders melt down the back towards the waist, and the arms remain soft.

Variation 2 – Plié Reach Series: From the end of #3, lower the gesture (right) leg to 45°, staying turned out in the hip joint, and connect the insides of the knees. Narrowing and hollowing to initiate the movement, curl the head and shoulders entirely off the floor, into the *Bowl of the Body* (see page 27). Lift the arms so that they are in a rounded oval parallel to the floor, hands behind the hamstrings. Extend the left leg out to 45°, externally rotating the hip joint to match the right leg. On count 1, inhale and slightly bend both knees while flexing the feet, creating a small demi plié in the legs. On count 2, extend both knees and point the feet, so that the legs reach back to the starting position; exhale on this action, increasing the narrowing and hollowing, and vocalize a long, deep, low-sounding "Huh." Do eight to sixteen repetitions. At the end, rotate parallel, bend both knees, and return to neutral stance in the legs, torso, and arms. The Plié Reach Series can also be done with the feet remaining pointed, and the big toes staying apart.

IMAGERY

Imagine on the Plié Reach Series that it is increased outward rotation that causes the knees to bend on the plié, so that the inner thighs revolve up towards the ceiling as they separate.

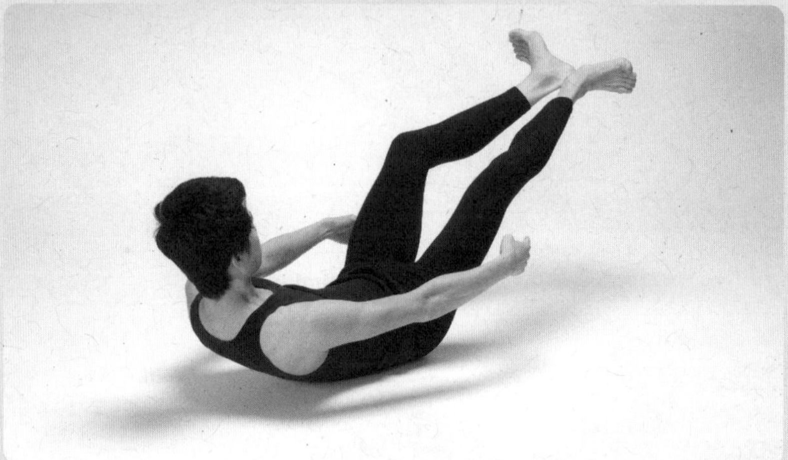

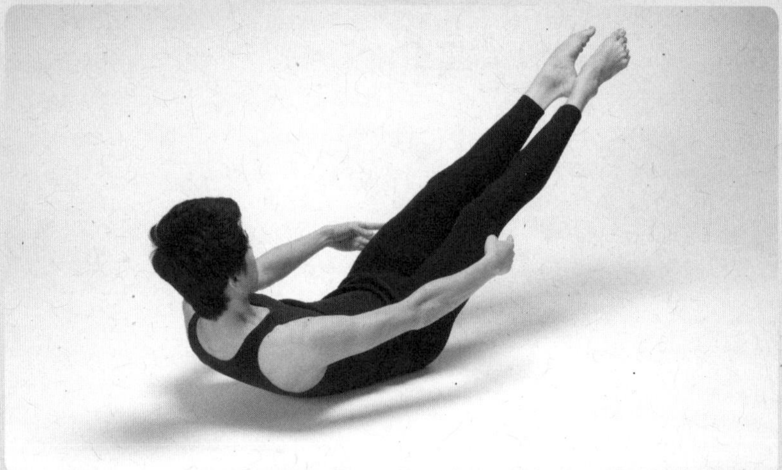

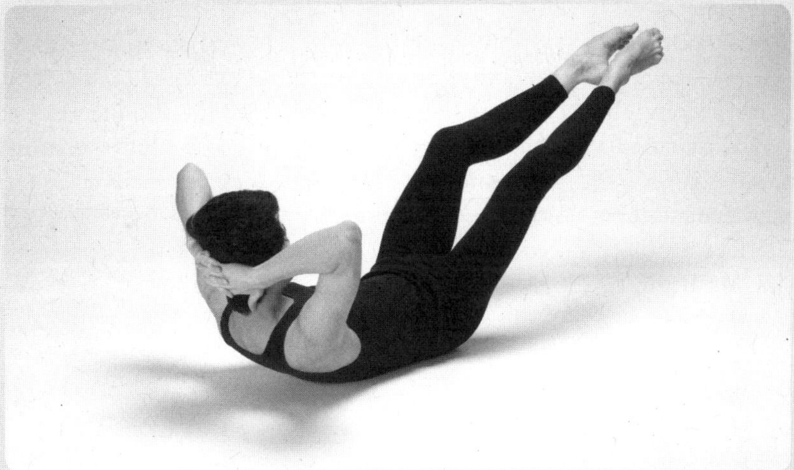

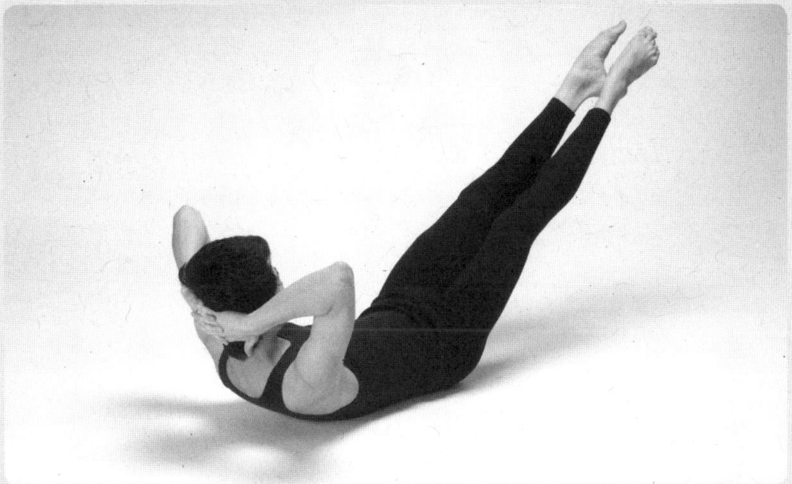

There are two advanced variations of plié reach.

Advanced Variation 1 – Outward/inward: This variation involves full rotational range of the hip joints. Begin with the same turned out demi plié action, keeping the feet pointed. Rotate the hips inward, and then extend. Repeat four times. Reverse the rotary action, so that the hips are turned in as the knees bend, and rotate out as the legs are extending. Repeat four times. Do another complete set: four times out to in, four times in to out. The feet remain pointed throughout this variation. Remember that the same breath rhythm applies, exhaling as the leg extends.

IMAGERY

During Advanced Variation 1 – Outward/inward, imagine that the toes are drawing circles in the space to assist in keeping the movement in the hips fluid.

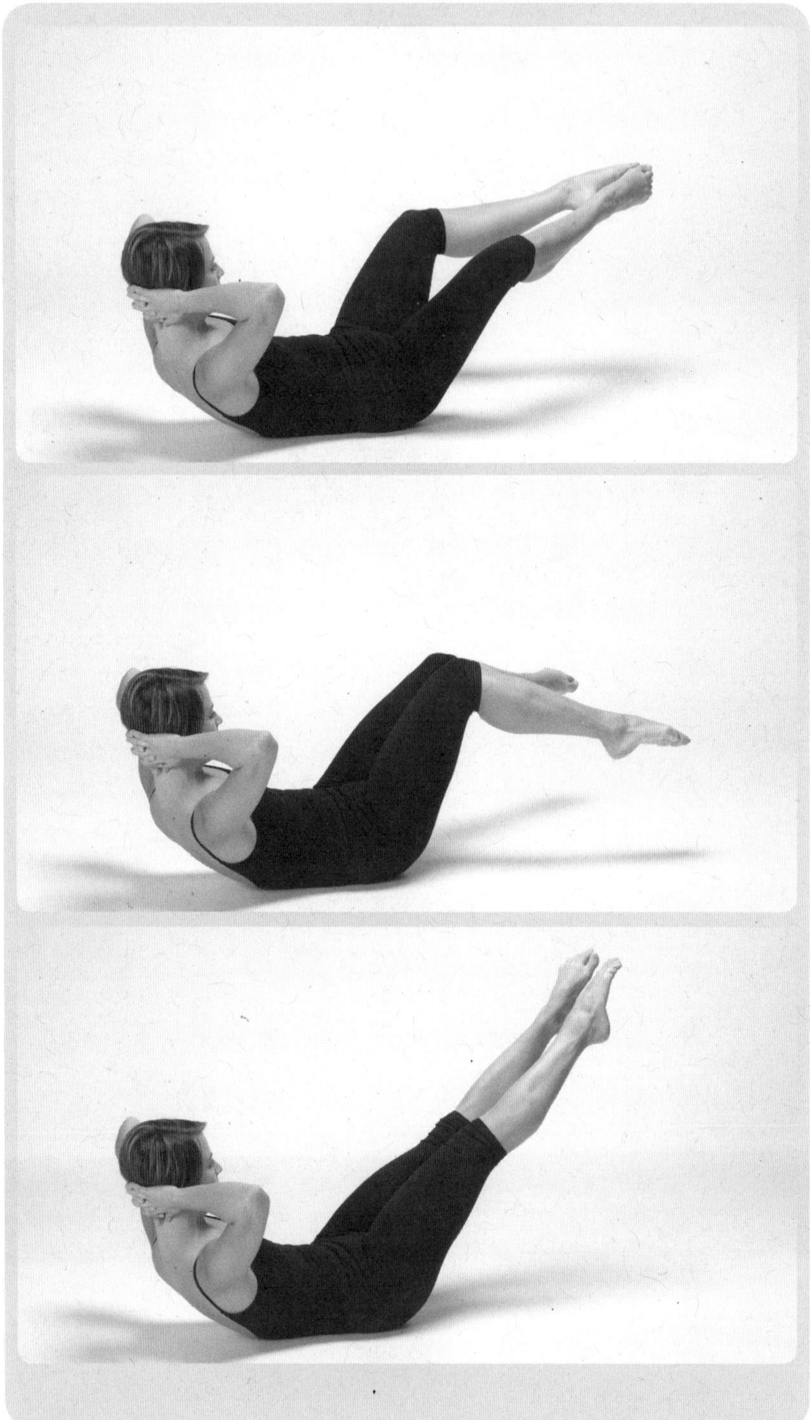

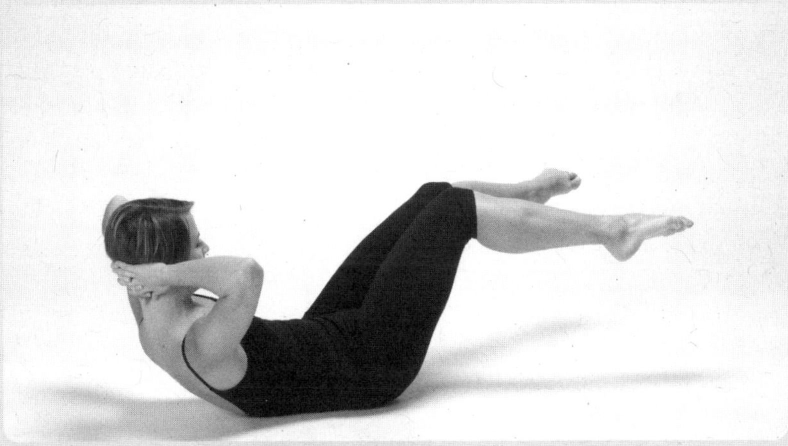

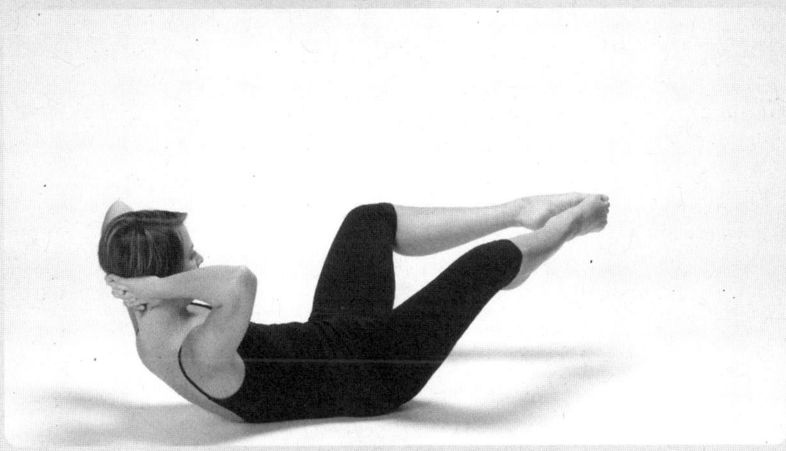

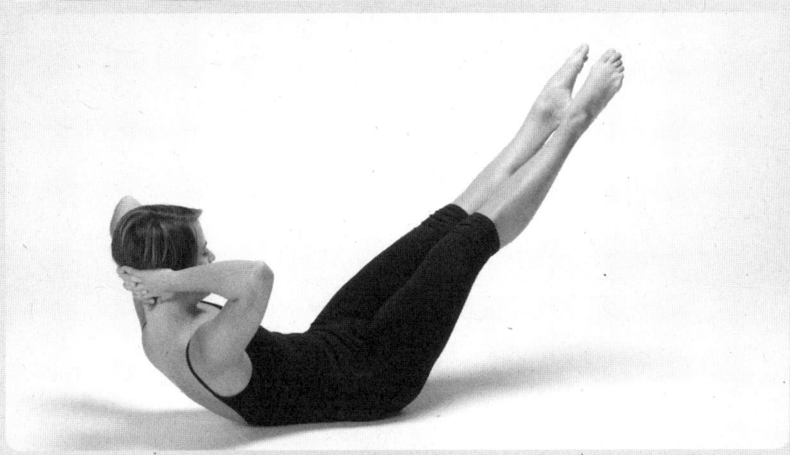

Advanced Variation 2 – Frog: Frog enhances core support with increased range of motion in the hips. Begin with the same turned out demi plié action, feet pointed. While maintaining the spatial placement of the thighs, extend the legs out. The legs can get wider, but not higher and, in fact, the closer the legs are to the floor, the more this challenges the core and abdominals. On the exhale, draw the legs together, keeping them extended, and flexing the feet. The feet point as the next plié is initiated. Do eight repetitions.

IMAGERY

During Advanced Variation 2 – Frog, imagine the legs moving easily through water.

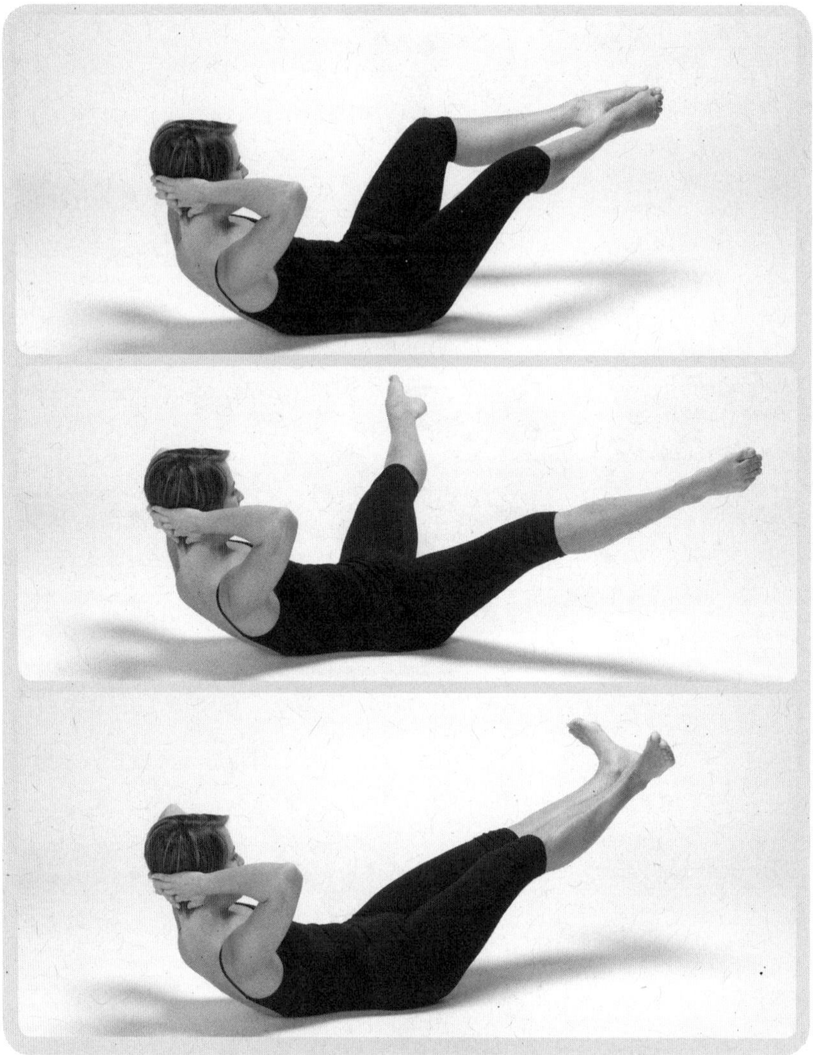

After this entire sequence, repeat everything on the left side.

The following variations can be added for the second side:

Arm variations: Instead of reaching the arms along the sides of the thighs, clasp the hands and place them gently at the back of the skull, with the elbows wide. This variation increases the workload for the abdominals. For advanced dancers, the arms can be placed in high fifth above the head, an even more challenging placement.

Foot variation: On the Plié Reach Series, the feet can remain pointed throughout the plié and extension. This variation challenges the dancer to experience the spatial reach of the legs without the change in foot position to assist.

Applications and Transfer to Standing and Travelling Work

The work in this series can be directly applied to standing and travelling in external rotation. By referring back to the sensory experience and images, dancers can be encouraged to externally rotate in stance utilizing the deep rotators, to maintain neutral pelvis in outward rotation, and to engage core support consistently. Additionally, the work encourages efficient use of balanced muscle function, and inhibits excess tension in large, superficial muscles and upper torso and arms.

The exercises in *Rotating In and Out* encourage the stabilization of the standing leg during active movement of the gesture leg. In particular, the use of the adductors is important because, in stance, the adductors contribute to external rotation and they help with balancing, particularly on one leg.

With *Lowering and Raising the Leg*, the added speed of the lifting leg assists with transfer to stance, as this dynamic emulates the action of a standing grand battement. Recalling the sensory experience of maintaining the sacrum on the floor can inhibit tucking under at the height of the battement.

The exercises in *Core Support with Moving Legs* contribute to the dancer's understanding and experience of "lift" or "pull-up" by imprinting the sensation of narrowing and hollowing, the lengthening throughout the spine, and energy out of the top of the head. When these images and kinesthetic sensations are brought to the attention in stance, it will encourage a lifted aesthetic without excess force. The integrated use of core support with leg action can contribute to injury prevention by ensuring that the core is engaged in vigorous movements such as jumps and jump landings, and partnering work.

Notes for Teachers

If the dancer is not able to maintain the foot/knee alignment in the rotation exercises, the teacher can put the dancers in pairs. One person can do the exercise while the partner creates a corridor with his or her arms, with one hand at each side of the foot lined up with the outer and inner knee. The foot and knee relationship should remain within this corridor.

The stretches of the hamstrings are done in parallel because it gives a more balanced stretch to this group of muscles. In particular, the lateral hamstrings tend to be tighter; stretching in parallel addresses this imbalance, as does as the crossed-over stretch (#3B).

There is some disagreement as to whether or not abdominal exercises should be done in spine flexion (the *Bowl of the Body*) or in neutral spine. The advantages to doing this work in flexion are a diminished chance of arching and straining the low back, particularly for dancers with weaker abdominals. Also, the action of staying in the undercurve encourages use of the lower abdominals and not just the upper rectus abdominus.

If a particular dancer cannot achieve the lift of the upper body off the floor for the *Touch Reach Series*, a simplified version is to have the dancer hold onto the legs underneath the hamstrings, and support the body weight. They should still actively use the breath, vocalization, and narrowing and hollowing with the leg movements. In all variations of the Touch Reach Series, watch for "touch poppers;" that is, dancers who snap the legs out in a sharp action, instead of a lengthening reach.

The teacher should make sure that the pliés in the Plié Reach Series are very small. The knees bend only enough to allow for a small amount of hip flexion, which releases the tension on the Y-ligament. This permits an increase in the possible external rotation at the hip. If the plié is large, it reduces the challenge to the abdominals by bringing the weight of the legs very close to the torso. In the version with the feet remaining pointed, make sure that the big toes do not touch each other in the plié phase.

One of the advantages of having the upper torso rolled up off the floor in the abdominal exercises is that the dancer can look at the lower abdominal area and watch it sink into the floor on each exhale. This visual feedback reinforces the sensory feedback. The teacher should make sure that the lumbar spine remains on the floor so that the dancer does not end up in a V-sit. As the dancers get stronger, the exercise can be made more challenging by lowering the legs closer to the floor, but at no time should the lumbar spine disengage from floor contact.

B – Sequencing from the Core to the Periphery

Purpose

The primary focus of this series is increased awareness and recruitment of the core, and how it engages with legwork. Each action is initiated by the narrowing and hollowing, and this support has to be maintained, especially on Variation 2. The second important idea is sequencing: The movements begin in the core, then the hamstrings engage, and finally, the gluteals engage at the highest point of the pelvis. This firing of the hamstrings is crucial for dancers to accomplish standing work, with efficient pelvic alignment without excess tension. Third, this series is designed to achieve balanced muscle function in the legs by increasing adductor recruitment, and reducing dependence on lateral musculature. It should be noted that variations of this exercise are commonly suggested by physiotherapists for back injury rehabilitation, and it is excellent for injury prevention as well. The final *Extensions from the Bridge* further engage the core support and leg control by placing all the weight on one leg, creating an additional challenge to the pelvis and spine alignment.

1) Exercise on 6 for the Spine

From neutral stance, separate the parallel legs to "open parallel" (knees and feet at the width of the ASIS bones), and bring the heels closer to the sitz bones. Arms are resting on the floor at the sides of the pelvis, and the spine and pelvis are in neutral alignment.

Variation 1 – Roll-Down: On count 1, exhale and initiate the movement of the spine with the undercurve (for reference, see page 25). In a continuous sequential action, on counts 2,3,4, roll the pelvis up off the floor, then the spine, until there is a long line from shoulders to knees, sometimes referred to as a bridge. The hips should be higher than the rib cage, which should remain soft, and the knees should remain parallel. Hold counts 5,6, inhaling during this sustained position. On the exhale, begin a sequential roll down for counts 1–4, starting at the top of the cervical spine, and reaching one vertebra at a time until the entire spine and sacrum have arrived on the floor. On 5,6, do an overcurve on the next exhale. Do three to four repetitions.

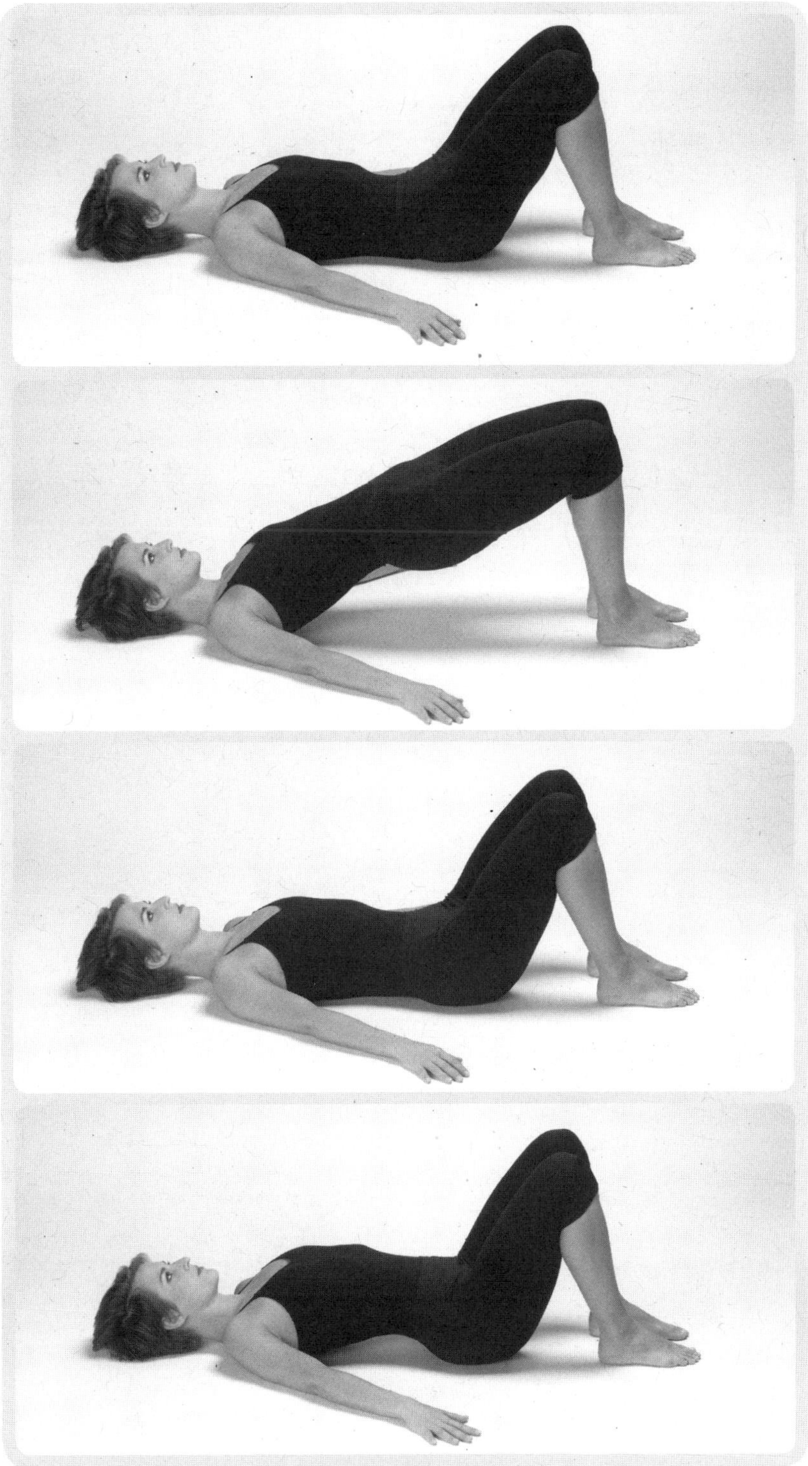

IMAGERY

For *Exercise on 6 for the Spine*, imagine squeezing a tennis ball between the knees. Keep this image going throughout the exercise. This image ensures that the space remains between the thighs, but the inner thighs are actively maintaining parallel, especially as the hips go higher. Use the narrowing and hollowing imagery for the initiating undercurve. On the roll-up, imagine that the neck and shoulders are softening and melting into the floor as the hips lift. On the roll-down, imagine tiny balloons filling with air between each vertebra as they lower one by one. On the final overcurve of Variation 1 of *Exercise on 6 for the Spine*, image the elastics from the pubic bone to lumbar spine elongating but staying taut.

Variation 2 – Arch Down: The first half of Variation 2 is the same as Variation 1. The recovery is a different pathway. Instead of the roll-down, reach the tailbone towards the floor and the heels, so that by count 4 the body has arrived in an elongated overcurve. On the inhale on counts 5,6, return the spine to neutral alignment. Do three to four repetitions.

IMAGERY

For Variation 2 of *Exercise on 6 for the Spine*, on the recovery to the floor (second 6 counts), imagine the tailbone diving off a high diving board and aiming for the heels. One can also envision the spine as a slinky, so that as the arch in the spine is created, the anterior surfaces of the vertebrae expand away from each other, and space is maintained between the posterior surfaces. At the end, in the return to neutral spine, send energy out of the top of the head and the tailbone to ensure maximum length.

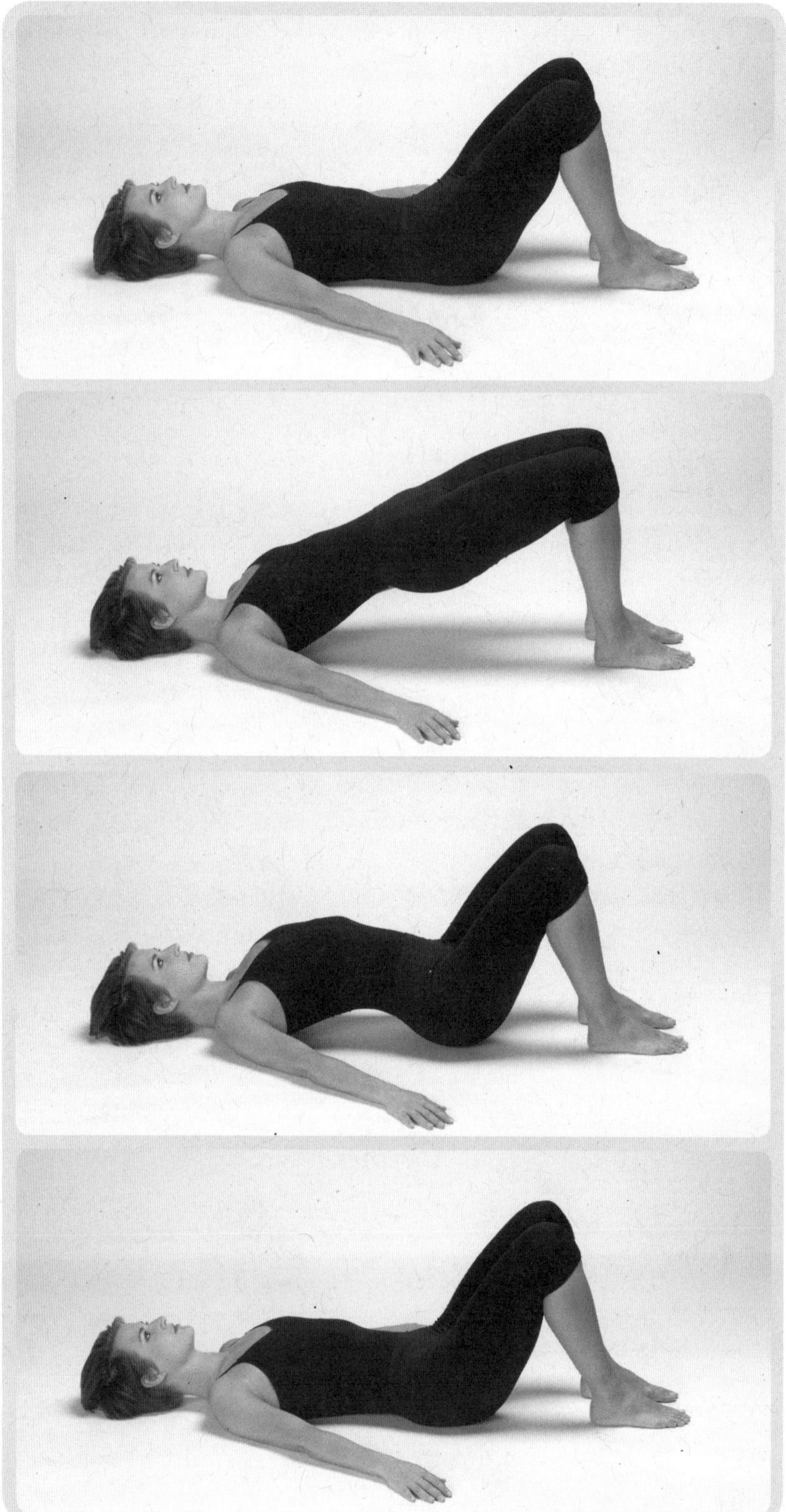

2) Extensions from the Bridge

At the end of either Variation 1 or Variation 2, do one additional roll-up to hold. From the bridge, extend the right knee without changing the level of the right thigh, so that the thighs remain in line. Bend the right knee to lower the foot back to the floor. Repeat on the left. Once again, extend the right knee without changing the level of the right thigh, keeping the thighs in line. Now reach the right leg higher, so that the foot reaches to the ceiling, without letting the hips drop. Lower the straight leg back in line with the left thigh, and then bend the right knee to lower the foot back to the floor. Repeat on the left.

Note: Other variations can be added to the second pair of lifts, such as flexing and pointing the foot that is to the ceiling, or rotating that leg externally and then back to parallel. One can even do an additional roll-down and roll-up with one leg reaching to the ceiling. For an advanced variation, once again extend the right knee without changing the level of the right thigh. Bend the right knee and lift the leg towards the ceiling, so that it comes to parallel attitude above the pelvis. Extend the right leg to the ceiling, lifting slightly higher in the pelvis. Slowly reach the leg in a long arc until the right heel touches the floor, keeping the leg extended and the pelvis at the same height. Bend the right knee and place the foot back to parallel stance. Repeat on the left side. At the end, do one more slow roll-down, bring the knees into the chest, hugging them with the arms, and say out loud, "Fabulous legs!"

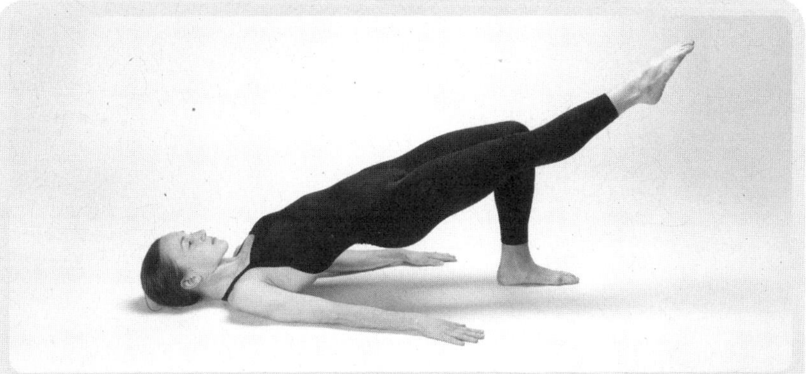

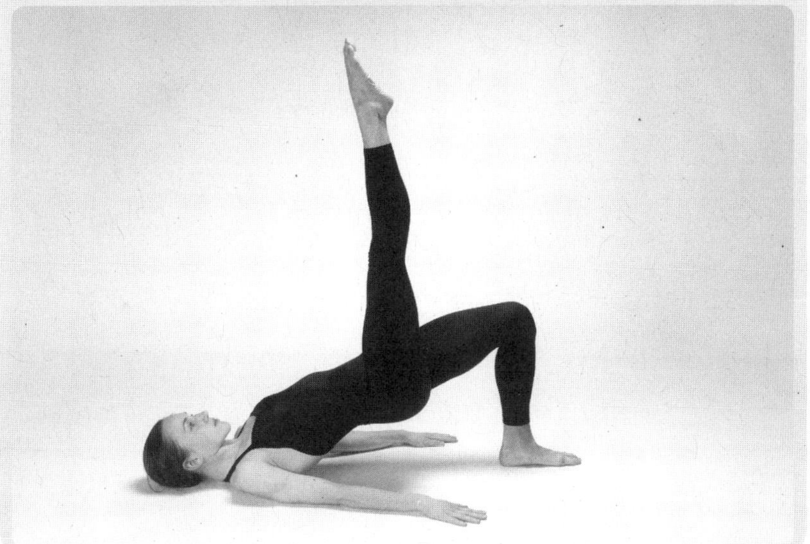

IMAGERY

For *Extensions from the Bridge*, imagine energy pouring out of the end of the foot on the knee extension. As the leg reaches to the ceiling, imagine that the foot is pulling the pelvis higher.

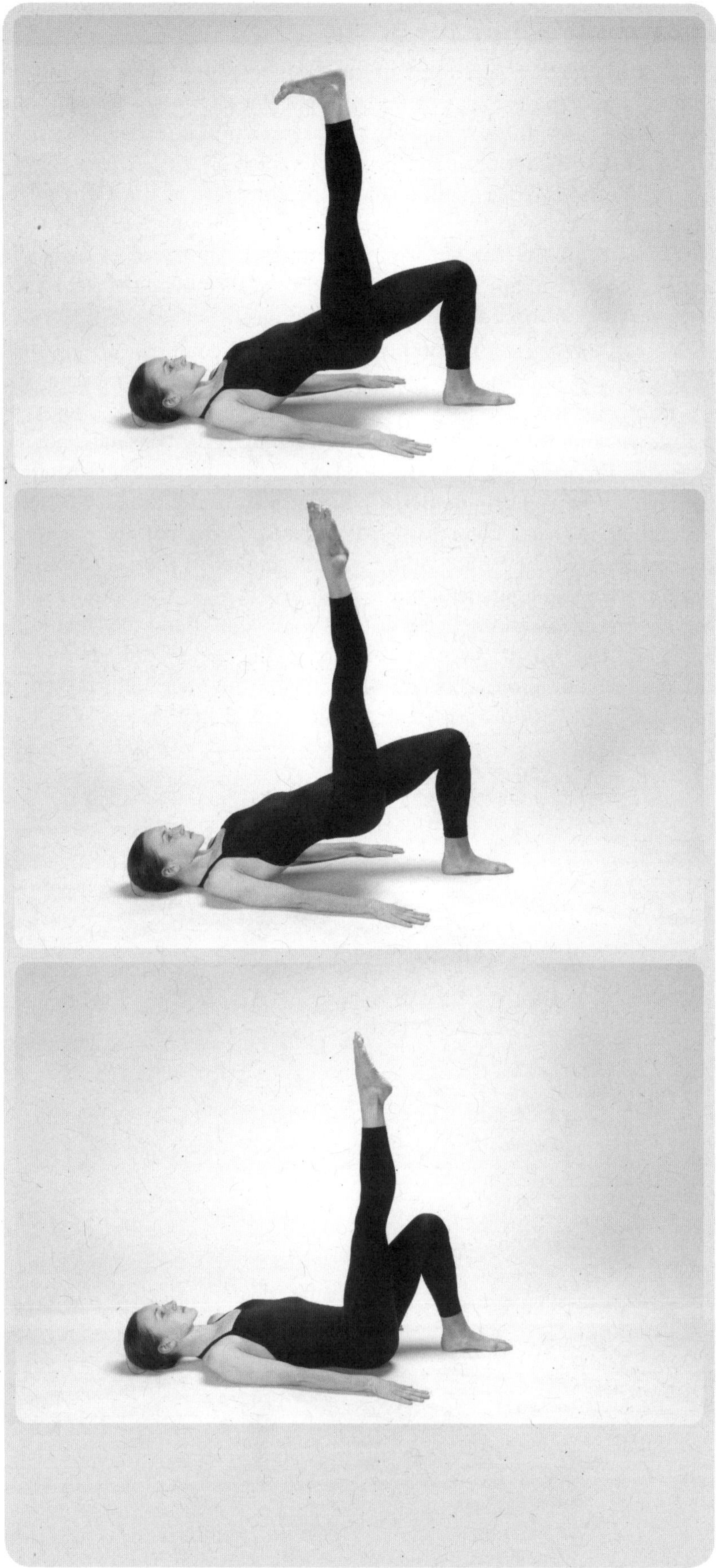

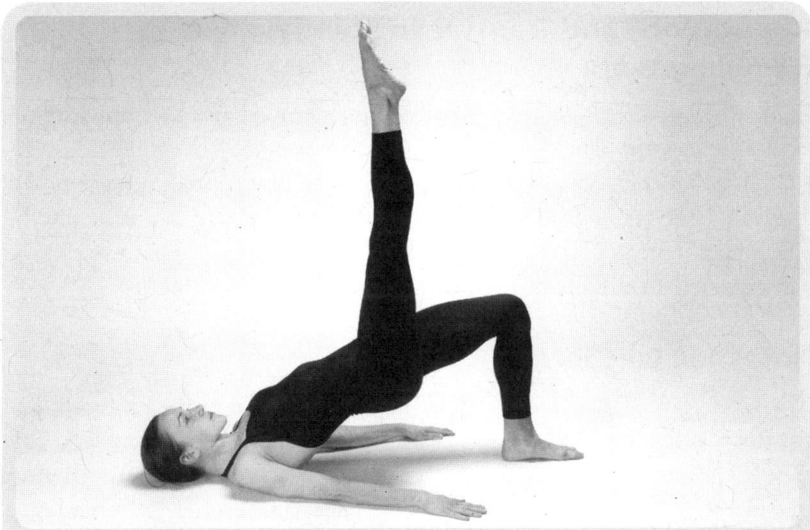

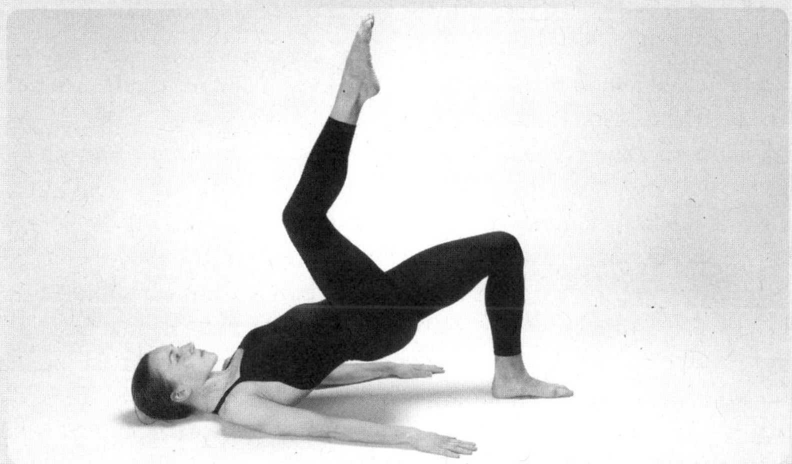

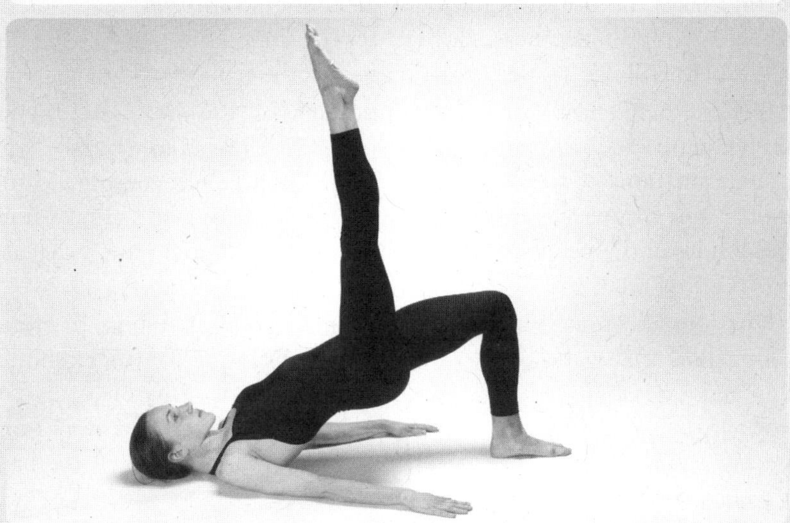

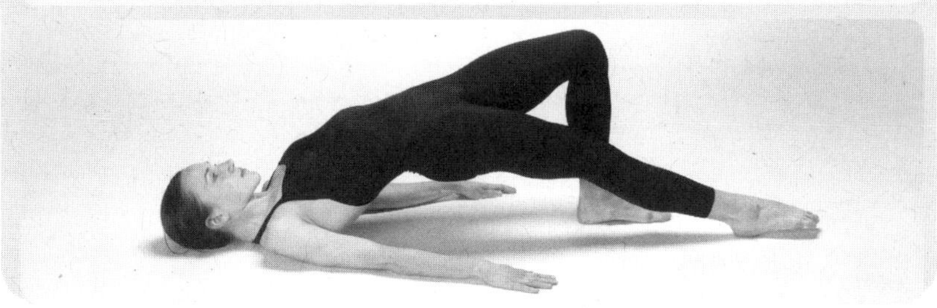

Applications and Transfer to Standing and Travelling Work

As described in this section, this counterbalanced use of core support (abdominals) and hamstrings is essential for efficiency in stance and travelling work. When dancers rely entirely on the gluteals to align the pelvis, it inhibits free use of the legs and moving through space. Additionally, the encouragement to engage the adductors also supports standing work, and eases tension in the quadriceps to maintain balance on the legs.

Notes for Teachers

It is important that the dancers be reminded to keep breathing and to continue releasing any excess tension in the neck and shoulders. The breath rhythm described above is essential to achieve the desired effect of each segment of the exercise. Additionally, the teacher can encourage continued breathing during the *Extensions from the Bridge*, as this portion has no prescribed breath counts.

The teacher should watch that the dancers maintain parallel distance between the feet, knees, and thighs throughout the exercise. Some dancers will allow the knees to fall open, and others will turnout from the feet as the series progresses. One way to establish this kinesthetic sensation is to teach this series in pairs. One person (the mover) lies on the back to do the exercise. The partner begins by making sure the mover's feet are parallel, moving the feet closer to the sitz bones. The feet should be as close as they can comfortably be, with no pain in the knees at any time. The partner places a fist between the knees, right between the medial condyles of the tibia. The mover is instructed to squeeze the fist as the partner provides verbal feedback and encouragement. Eventually the partner takes the fist away, but the dancer should imagine that there is still a fist or an object there. This can also be done using tennis balls, but tennis balls will not correct foot alignment or give feedback!

While there may be some adjustment of the head and pelvis placement in the final counts of Variation 2 (the return to neutral), large accommodations generally indicate that the dancer has compressed the lumbar area in the overcurve coming down. The teacher can take hold of the sides of the pelvis during this movement, and guide the spine into an elongated recovery.

Two modifications: First, if the hips cannot go high enough to create a long line, it may be due to hip flexor tightness. The dancer should be given a flexibility exercise for this area, to be described later in this program. Second, if there is pain in the knees, move the feet away from the sitz bones. In extreme cases it may be necessary to widen the base as well.

C - Releasing the Hips for Second Position

Purpose

This series is designed to increase range of motion in the hips for second position work (sitting, développé, grand battement) through both muscular stretching and neuromuscular release of tension patterns. Additionally, it gives the dancer information about the correct placement of the legs in second position, and sensory feedback from the floor about neutral spine and pelvis alignment when the legs are in second position. The series is designed to minimize superficial muscle use, while encouraging deeper muscles to support the movement.

1) Jiggles

There are two variations of the *Jiggles*, "outies" and "uppies." From the position of hugging the knees into the chest, gently open the legs apart, keeping the knees relaxed and folded. Place the hands on the inner thighs right above the inside of the knee joint. Using the hands to gently pulse the legs, do a quick jiggling action that opens the inner thighs outward. Change the hands so that they are placed around the outside of the thighs and on the shins, just below the knee. Continue the jiggling action, but now the direction is upward towards the shoulders (not inward). One way to view the directions of this action is that the "outies" assist in widening the legs in second position extensions, and the "uppies" address the height of the leg in second position extensions. The timing should be brisk, and one can do sixteen quick counts of "outies," then sixteen quick counts of "uppies." Keep alternating for three to four sets.

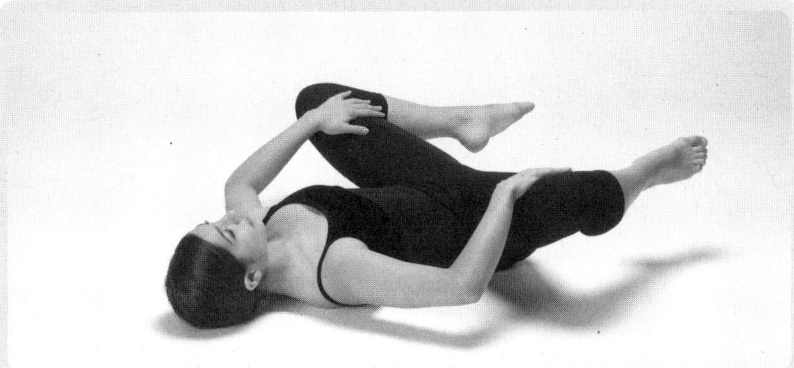

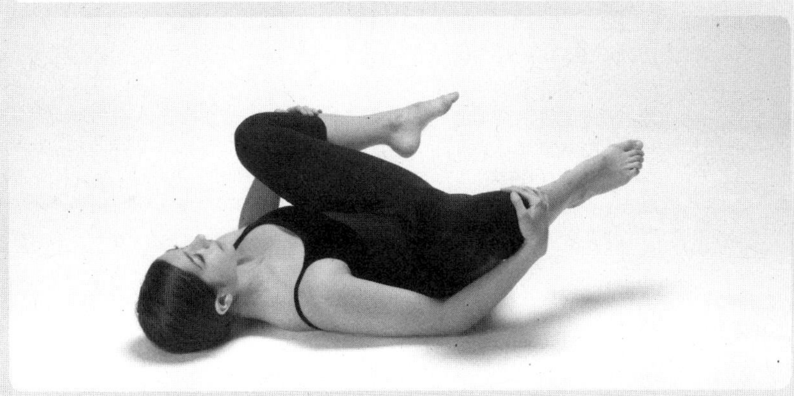

IMAGERY

For *Jiggles*, imagine that the hips have no muscles, and the hands are pulsing the femoral heads in jelly-coated sockets. The sacrum should still be weighted on the floor, so that the pelvis does not rock in any direction during the *Jiggles*. The action is entirely in the socket. Visualize the playful quality babies have when they move their legs around with their hands. Imagine flopping feet on the ends of the legs.

2) Second Position Extensions on 3

At the end of the *Jiggles*, begin rubbing the inner thighs vigorously and slowly extend the legs to second position. Keep the hands on the inner thighs, holding the legs and supporting their weight to minimize tension in the hip flexors; these muscles should remain as soft and passive as possible. From extended second, bend the knees and flex the feet so that the legs are in side attitude. On a count of 3, exhale and extend the legs out to second as the feet point sequentially, "heel, ball of the foot, toes," and then reverse the action on the next 3, inhaling and bending the knees again as the feet flex, "toes, ball of the foot, heel." Repeat this action four to eight times.

IMAGERY

For *Second Position Extensions on 3*, imagine air or light pouring out of the feet as they extend into the space. See the feet reaching further away from the pelvis, causing the knees to extend. Imagine the tailbone reaching into the floor to avoid tucking under (posterior pelvic tilt). On the plié, imagine a softening and folding of the ankle, knee, and hip joints. Reinforce the image of narrowing and hollowing to avoid bracing and tightening in the trunk muscles.

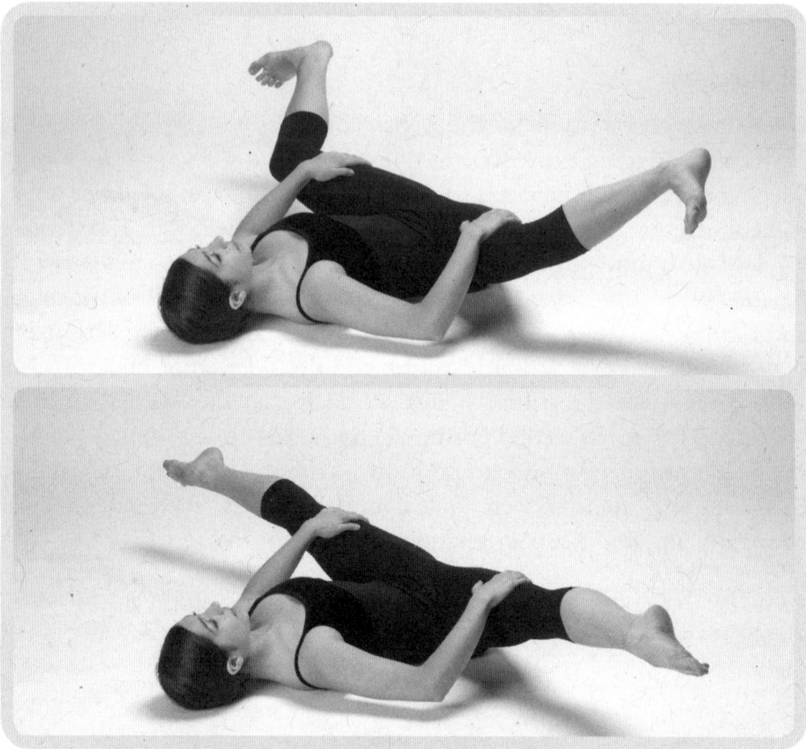

3) Second Position Stretch

After the last extension, relax the feet and soften the knees, remaining in open second position for a passive stretch. Continue holding the weight of the legs with the hands, and focusing on the release of tension in the hips. After about thirty seconds, gently and slowly fold the legs into the chest, place the feet onto the floor, slide the legs out long, and rest.

IMAGERY

For *Second Position Stretch*, imagine the legs very heavy and dropping towards the earth. Use the breath to assist in relaxation, imagining the air filling the hip joints on the inhale, and taking the tension away on the exhale.

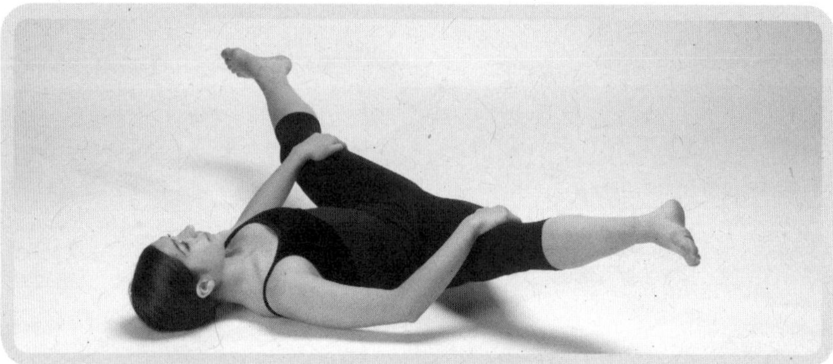

Applications and Transfer to Standing and Travelling Work

This series directly applies to standing work using second position leg gestures. The *Jiggles* allow dancers to experience the articulation of the femur in the hip socket freely, so that they have a reference point of sensory information when they stand and do side extensions. This work also promotes the long line of the leg, and creates a sense of "energy" out of the foot in gesture work.

Notes for Teachers

Make sure that the dancers are performing a loose, non-muscular action in the *Jiggles*, and that the feet are relaxed and flopping. This exercise triggers a laughter response, so do not be surprised if the dancers giggle and laugh throughout the *Jiggles*.

Modify both the *Second Position Extensions on 3* and the passive stretch exercises for those dancers with less flexibility. The legs should be on the torso side of the pelvis in relation to the line of gravity, so if the dancers cannot straighten the legs while maintaining that relationship, the legs can stay bent at the end of the reach. As the dancer gains more flexibility, the legs can reach further until arriving at full extension.

Throughout this series, check for ease in the neck and shoulders, and that the breathing remains even and fluid. Encourage the dancers to minimize tension in the thighs through the use of the imagery and the breath.

The legs can turn out fully, as long as it does not encourage rolling/tucking in the pelvis.

As the dancers become more advanced in this series, they can add the concept of gradual increase in leg height; that is, as the legs bend, slightly lift the femurs in the direction of the shoulders (staying wide), and as the legs extend, maintain that new femoral range.

PART THREE
FLEXIBILITY SERIES

Opening Remarks

The goal of this entire section is improved flexibility and range of motion. There are several reasons to encourage flexibility in certain muscle groups. First, there is the release of tension that builds up with repetitive movement (such as the outward rotators of the hips). Second, there is muscle balancing; that is, addressing antagonist muscle groups that are inhibiting easeful action at the joint due to strength/flexibility imbalances (such as hamstrings and quadriceps). Third, there is lengthening of muscles that inhibit good alignment (such as the hip flexors). Fourth, there is injury prevention (such as adequate flexibility in the calf muscles to allow for good shock absorbency in jump landings). Fifth, there are aesthetic reasons to have excellent range of motion in dance practice (such as stretching the legs in second position).

Flexibility should not exceed strength and coordination to the point that joint stability is compromised. This series has been placed at this point in the program to promote the range of motion needed for easeful execution of the exercises still to come. For hypermobile dancers, this section can be skipped. Dancers needing additional flexibility should be encouraged to do this section regularly. This section can be done as a group of exercises at this point in the C-I Training program, or it can be moved to the very end. If a class is later in the day or evening, and the dancers do not have to dance vigorously after the C-I Training, then it is very effective to do the flexibility series at the end. These stretches can also be interspersed throughout the program at the discretion of the teacher. For the sitting stretches, it is useful to provide a pillow or towel for less flexible dancers to sit on, to elevate the hips above the legs. If this adaptation is still uncomfortable and ineffective for less flexible dancers, they can do lying versions of the stretches, using a theraband or towel to support the limbs. Generally, these stretches should be maintained for a minimum of thirty seconds each. This can be adjusted at the teacher's discretion. You will notice that some of the exercises have progressions to be done in sequence, while others have variations. Select the appropriate one(s) for the class or individual.

If the Flexibility Series, in total or in part, is done in the middle of the C-I Training program, return to the floor after the final stretch, and lie on the back to prepare for the next section. If the flexibility series is done at the end of the C-I Training program, come to a parallel demi plié with the torso hanging forward, roll slowly up the spine on the inhale, and take some time to find easeful, standing alignment. Imagery for this finish will be given at the end of the program.

Purpose

Each of these stretches targets different muscle groups for a variety of reasons. *Sitting with Folded Legs* targets the deep muscles in the posterior hip joint and the spine for aesthetic range of motion. Additionally, if the hips are tight, the surrounding muscles will overwork to gain higher extensions, causing possible fatigue injuries. *Sitting with the Soles of the Feet Together* aids in increased range in the muscles that inhibit outward rotation, thus potentially assisting in improved range of motion in this important hip movement for dancers. *Hanging over Extended Legs* targets the hamstrings, and assists in improved range of motion for legwork to the front; some dancers will also experience release of back tension. *Pretzel* stretches the external rotators of the hip, a muscle group that is used excessively in dance; tightness in these muscles can lead to discomfort and even nerve impingement in extreme cases. *Sitting in Second Position* targets the hip adductors, as well as the medial hamstrings, improving range of motion in second position extensions. Side-bending variations also address tightness in the side muscles of the torso, important for use of the body in contemporary work in particular. All the variations in *Quadriceps Variations* are for the quadriceps group and are designed to focus particularly on the lateral quadriceps (vastus lateralis), which often are tighter than the medial muscles. Tightness in these lateral muscles is a contributing factor to many knee problems in dancers, including patellar femoral syndrome. *Hip Flexor Lunge* is another essential stretch for dancers, and is for the flexors of the hip. If these muscles are tight, they contribute to "swayback" (anterior pelvic tilt) and can cause many problems for dancers including inefficient use of turnout, low back pain and injuries, and possible psoas injuries. Length in the hip flexors is essential for achieving neutral pelvis in stance and dynamic motion. *Mountain* targets the calf muscles, another highly used group in dance during relevés, pointe work, and jumps. Tightness in the calves is a contributing factor in shin splints and related injuries. *Standing and Hanging* deals again with hamstring flexibility and, for some dancers, spine flexibility.

IMAGERY

In general, stretching is most beneficial when combined with release of tension through the use of breath and imagery, rather than by using external force. This method teaches the dancer how to diminish tension that is inhibiting range of motion, in addition to encouraging flexibility in the muscles. A useful image with the breath is to imagine the area of tension filling with the inhale and the tension leaving the body with the exhaled air, or a sense of the body emptying. Because the idea of release is so essential to this approach to flexibility training, it is suggested that all muscles and joints be in a relaxed state, rather than, for example, trying to straighten the leg and point the feet during hamstring stretching.

1) Sitting with Folded Legs (with Variations)

(A) Sit up and fold the legs in front of the body, with the right leg closer to the body and the left leg on the outside. Slowly exhale and roll down until the body is hanging over the legs and the arms are relaxed on the floor in front of the legs. (B) Move the torso so that the forehead is over the right (inside) knee. Reach the left arm along the floor on the downstage right diagonal, melting the left shoulder towards the floor. This variation will increase the stretch for the left side of the back and, for some dancers, the left hip. (C) On the exhale, return back to the centre position, sinking the weight deeper into the floor. Slowly inhale and roll up. (D) Extend the left leg out along the floor directly in front of the left hip, adjusting the right leg so that the bottom of the right foot is against the left inner thigh. Exhale and hang over the long leg. Slowly inhale and roll up. Bring both legs forward, shake them out easily, and repeat everything on the second side.

IMAGERY

For *Sitting with Folded Legs*, imagine the hip sockets softening and folding, letting any tension in the hips and spine melt away with the breathing. See both thighs dropping and sinking towards the floor, as though they are becoming heavier. Imagine the head is a heavy weight, falling into the floor, opening the neck and spine. For the diagonal reach (B), imagine the opposite hip (i.e., the left hip if the torso is over the right thigh) dropping more deeply into the floor, and the side of the body elongating. For one leg extended (D), see the back of the thigh expanding, like cheese melting on the floor. For the roll-up at the end, imagine that there is a small balloon between each of the vertebrae, so that the spine is very tall as the body returns to vertical.

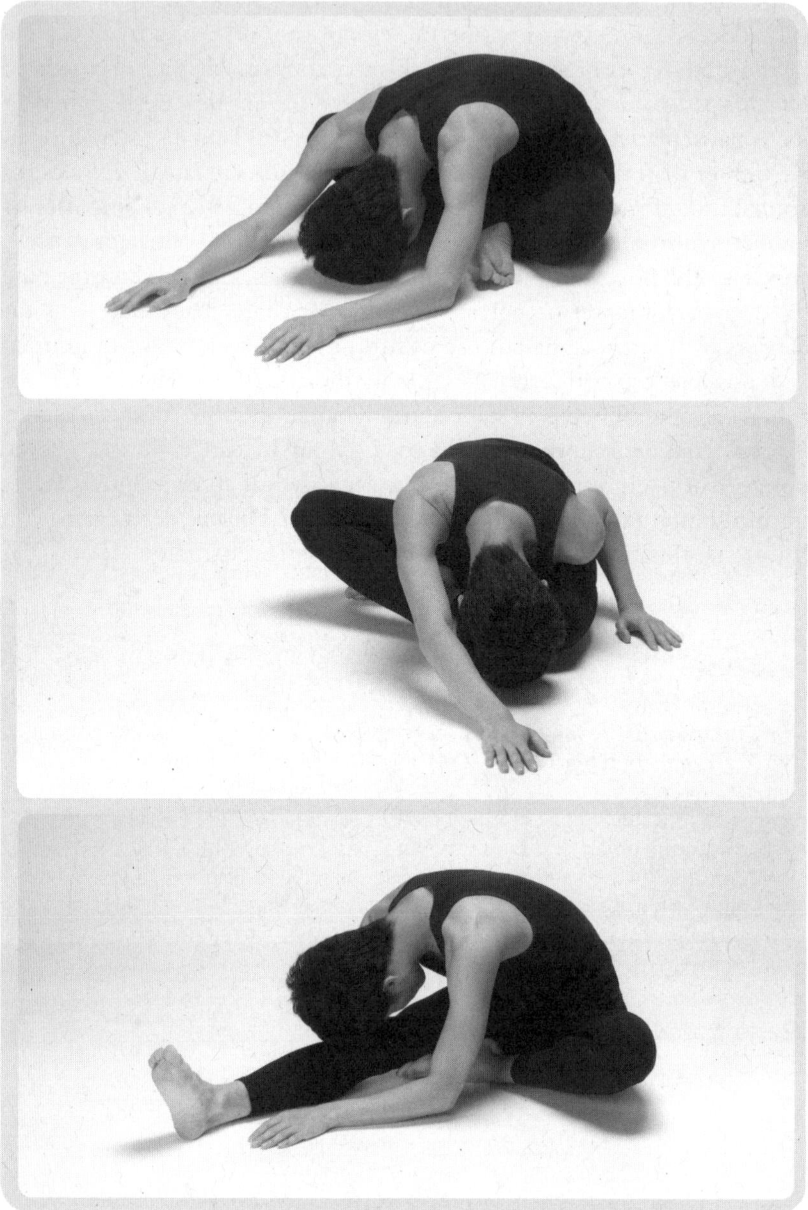

2) Sitting with the Soles of the Feet Together (Diamond)

(A) Clasp the hands at the back of the head. On the inhale, lengthen the spine and expand the elbows wide; on the exhale, roll down the spine until the torso is hanging over the feet, elbows hanging towards the floor. Release the arms gently to the floor. (B) Place the hands at the ankles and the elbows on the inner thighs, and gently press the legs towards the floor. Release the arms. Slowly inhale and roll up. Bring both legs forward and shake them out easily.

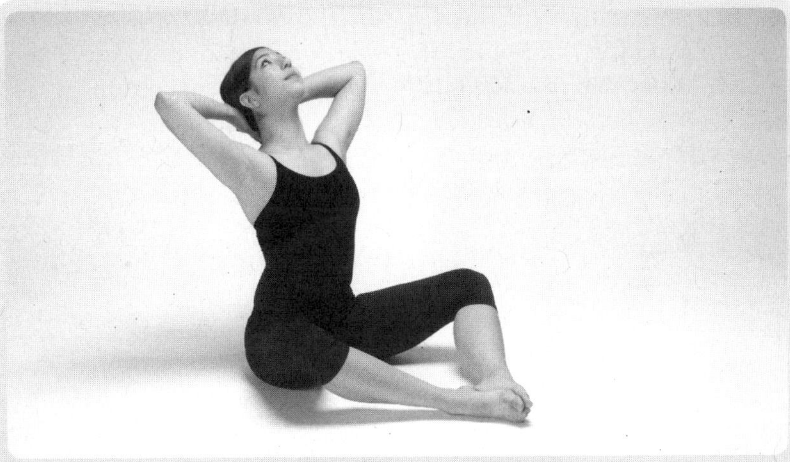

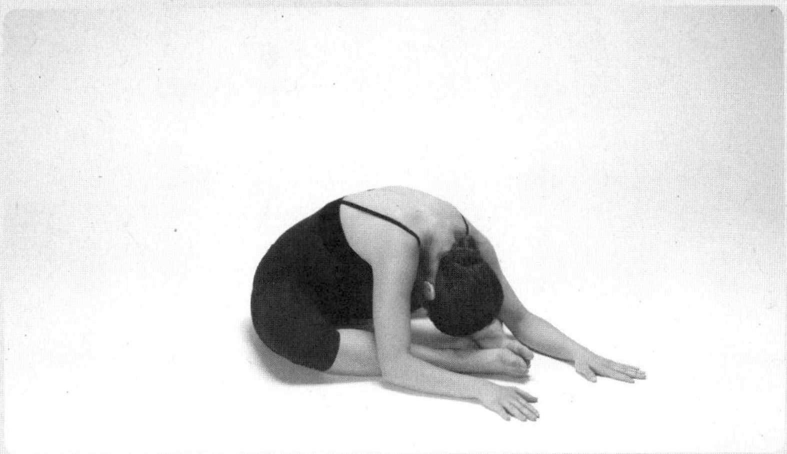

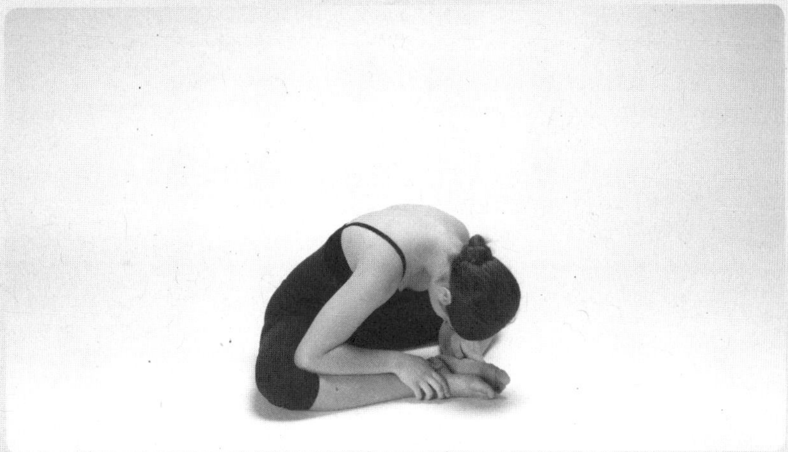

IMAGERY

For *Sitting with the Soles of the Feet Together*, the same images can apply to the hang over the Diamond. When pressing the thighs open, imagine that the thighs are yielding and sinking to the floor, rather than resisting the pressure (for variation B). This press must be gentle so that the legs do not contract reflexively. See the sitz bones as heavy and attached to the floor, so the pelvis does not roll forward.

3) Hanging over Extended Legs

(A) Sit with the legs extended in front of the body. Clasp the hands at the back of the head. On the inhale, arch the upper spine and expand the elbows wide; on the exhale, roll down the spine until the torso is hanging over the long legs. With the hands remaining clasped behind the head, allow the weight of the arms to assist in stretching out the muscles of the spine. (B) Release the arms gently to the floor. Elongate the back so that it is extended into neutral spine in a forward diagonal over the thighs. Flex the feet and take hold of them either over the top or around the arches. (C) Release the feet, drop the torso over the thighs once more, sinking the weight deeper, and allow the arms to relax by the sides of the legs. Slowly inhale and roll up. Shake the legs out easily and rock them through inward and outward rotation in a gentle rolling action.

IMAGERY

For *Hanging over Extended Legs*, allow the weight of the arms to add to the weight of the head and spine, and see the entire upper torso spilling onto the thighs. For the flat back variation (B), imagine the energy of the spine reaching out the top of the head on the diagonal like a beam of light.

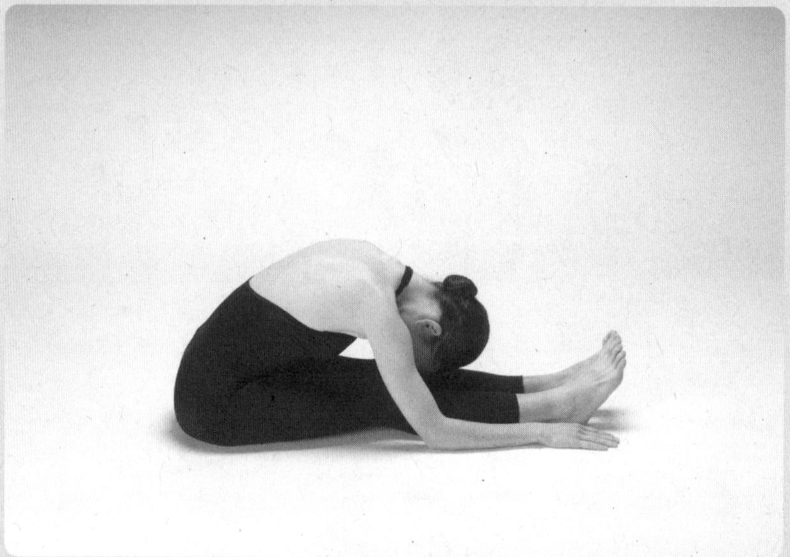

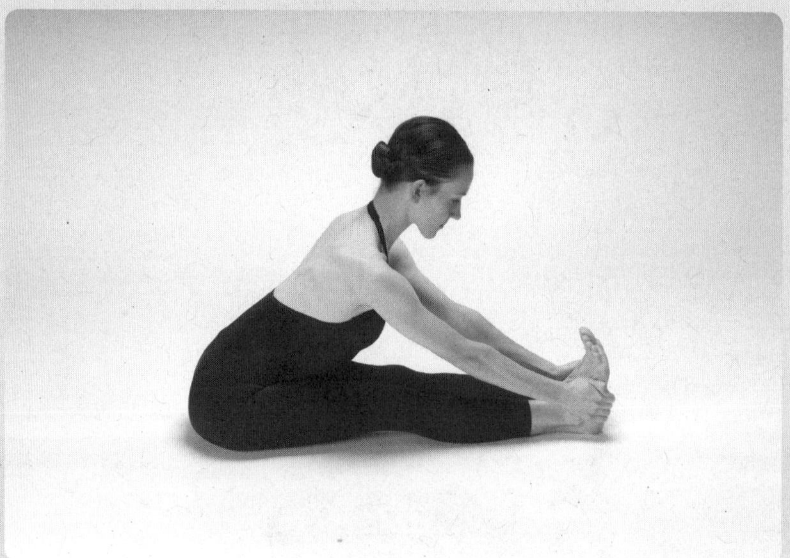

4) Pretzel

(A) Sit with the left leg folded on the floor turned out, and cross the right leg over, placing that foot on the floor near the left thigh. Turn the body to face the right knee and, using the left arm, draw the knee towards the left shoulder, trying to keep both sitz bones on the floor. Imagine the right hip gently sliding back and dropping down to the floor as the right knee and left shoulder come closer together. (B) Once this stretch is comfortable, a more intense variation can be done by taking hold of the left knee with the left hand, spiraling the spine around to the back, and staying very long and extended in the torso.

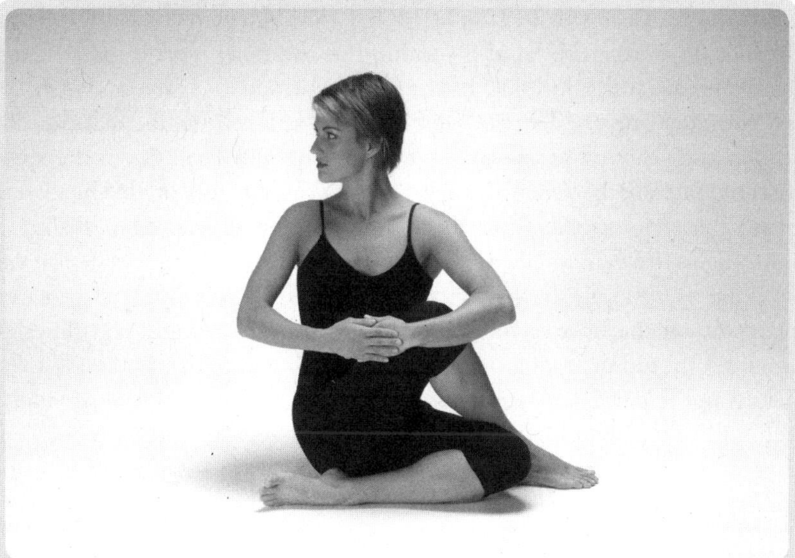

IMAGERY

For *Pretzel*, see the held thigh folding into the shoulder, while imagining the hip socket of that leg creasing deeper, and gently reaching down to the floor and to the back wall. With each inhale, imagine the spine elongating and growing taller.

5) Sitting in Second Position

(A) Sit with the legs in open second position with the knees relaxed but pointing to the ceiling, and the feet relaxed. Wrap the left arm behind the waist, palm facing away from the body, using this arm to keep the left shoulder wide. Place the right hand on the floor behind the right leg, and next to the right hip. On the exhale, release the head to the right and roll down the spine to the right side, keeping the focus straight ahead. The torso will be hanging just behind the legs, in line with the pelvis. (B) Release the left arm from the waist and slowly reach it up to the ceiling on the inhale; on the exhale, reach the arm to the opposite wall, fingers pointing towards the right side of the room, palm facing down. Keep the arm long and extended. (C) Circle the arm over the top and to the side so that the hand is reaching to the floor next to the left hip. Maintain the full side bend to the right, and create space between the left shoulder and the left ear. Slowly inhale and roll up. Repeat the side stretch and selected variations on the left side. (D) Roll down the spine directly forward between the legs, starting at the top of the head, and bring the arms to the floor in front of the body. Maintain the knees pointing to the ceiling. Slowly inhale and roll up. (E) A final variation can be done by rotating the spine to face the right leg, and keeping the left sitz bone on the floor. Roll down and hang over the right leg. The left shoulder should drop down and be level with the right shoulder. Slowly inhale and roll up. Repeat facing the left leg. Transition: Place the hands behind the body, and gently bring the legs together. Shake the legs out easily and rock them through inward and outward rotation in a gentle rolling action.

IMAGERY

For *Sitting in Second Position*, in each of the side-bending and rotating variations, imagine the opposite hip (i.e., the left hip when hanging to the right) sinking towards the floor, and that knee pointing to the ceiling. For the arm wrapped at the waist and the arm reaching down to the side (variations A and C), imagine the distance from the ear to the shoulder expanding (if side bending right, this would be the left ear and shoulder). For the body directly forward (D), see the legs falling open wider as the body weight sinks to the floor, again keeping both knees facing the ceiling.

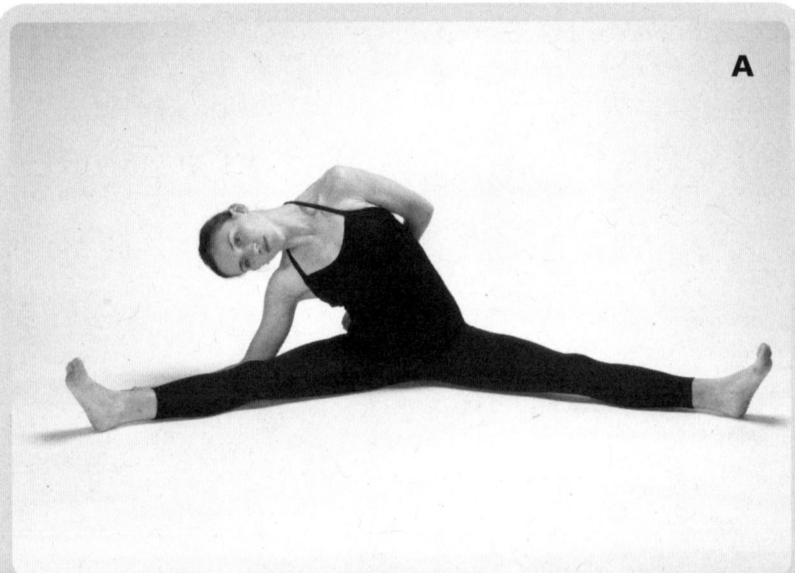

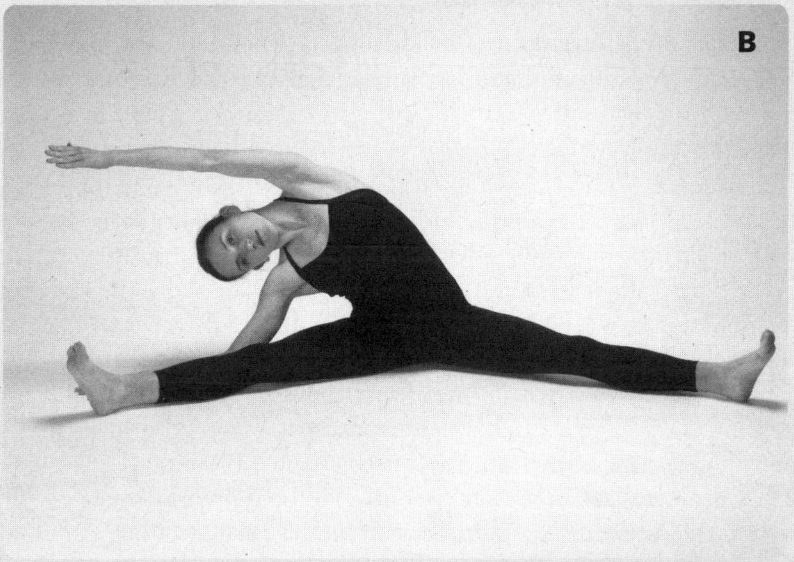

B

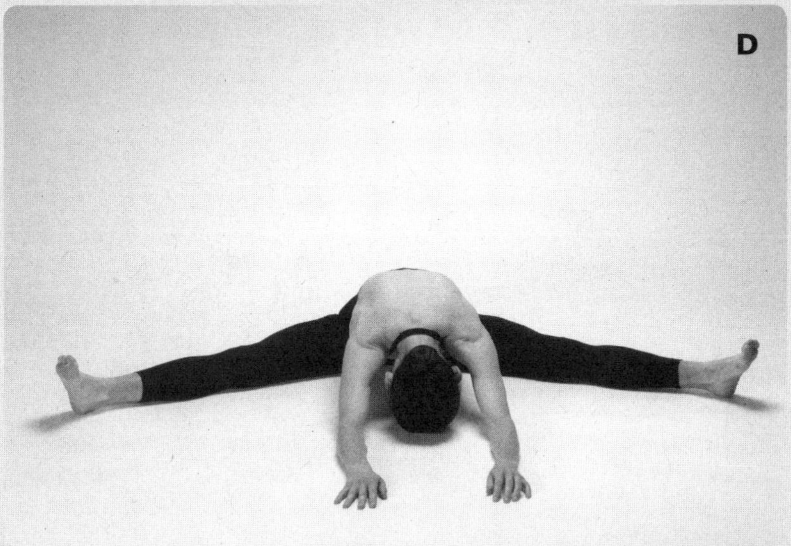

D

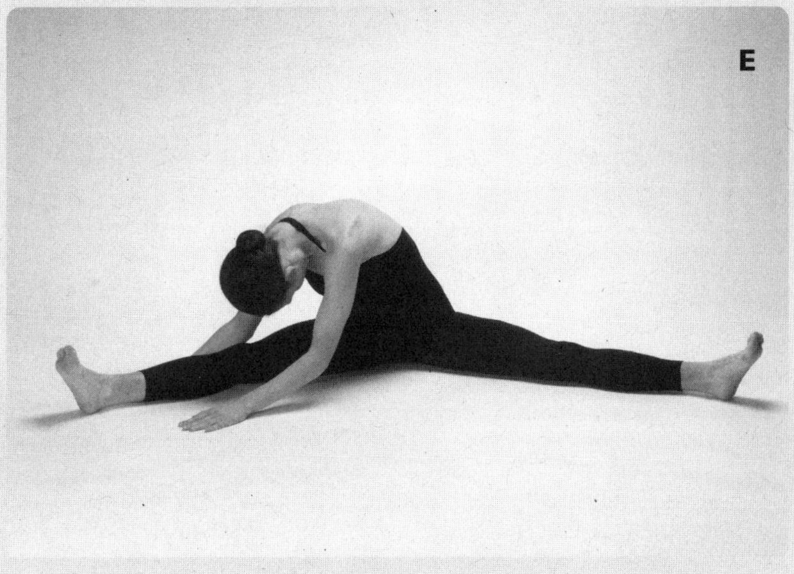

E

6) Quadriceps Variations

There are several variations of quadriceps stretches. The most important goal is for the dancer to find a version that successfully stretches this muscle group without strain or discomfort to the knee joint. Select one of the following options:

Variation 1 – Side-Lying: Lie on the right side of the body, supporting the head on the right arm. Fold both knees in front of the body with the feet directly under the pelvis. Move the left leg, so that by increasing the flexion in the left hip, the knee rests on the floor above the right leg. Slide the right leg back behind the pelvis, and bend the knee so that you can take hold of the right ankle with the left hand. Maintain the pelvic alignment so that the left hip is directly above the right hip, rather than allowing the front of the pelvis to roll towards the floor. Also, maintain the neutral alignment of the spine and pelvis so that the lumbar spine does not arch. Gently draw the right foot towards the right hip. To increase the stretch, slide the right knee further behind the pelvis without disturbing the alignment of the spine. Slowly release the foot, relax onto the back, and repeat on the second side.

IMAGERY

For Variation 1 – Side-Lying, imagine the body lying on a balance beam, so that the arm on the floor, the ribs, and the pelvis are all maintained in a long line.

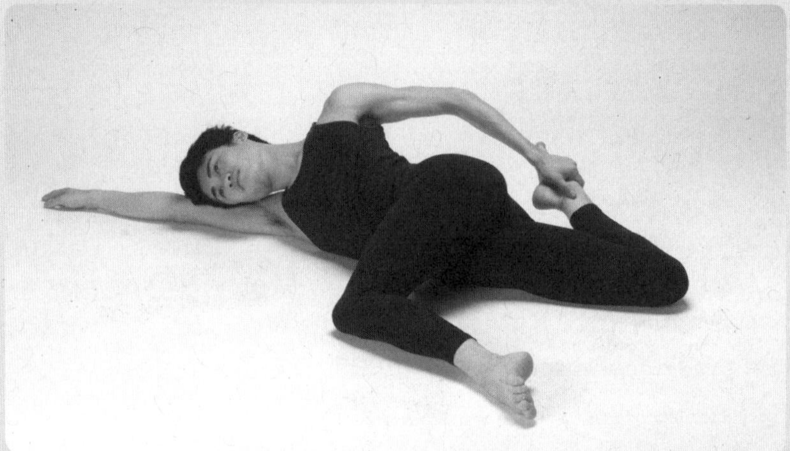

Variation 2 – Sitting on the Heels: Begin by sitting on the heels with the hands on the floor behind the feet for support. Bring the left foot forward and place it in stance near the right thigh. Using the hands, adjust the angle and height of the pelvis until a stretch in the right quadriceps is felt. For an added stretch to the quadriceps muscle, walk the left foot out to the side without changing the facing of the pelvis, and slide the right knee along the floor towards the left foot. Gently unfold the legs, and repeat on the second side.

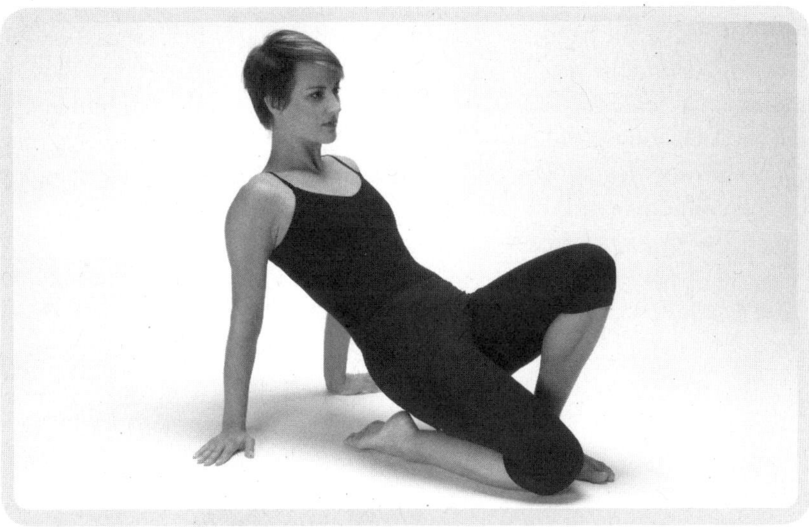

Variation 3 – Back-Lying: Fold the right leg and fully inward rotate the hip, placing the knee on the floor. Bring the right foot next to the right hip, with the knee in line with the midline of the body, not opening out to the side. The right foot should be pointed (not flexed), with the top of the foot facing down to the floor. This is important as it minimizes torque at the knee. The left leg is extended forward in front of the left hip. Initiate the stretch by placing the hands behind the body, and moving the pelvis so that the sacrum is reaching towards the floor (in the direction of posterior pelvic tilt). For many dancers, this position will provide an adequate stretch. If the dancer does not yet experience a quadriceps stretch, the spine can continue moving towards the floor until the dancer is resting on the elbows and, eventually, lying down. The spine should remain in neutral (not in excessive lumbar arch) and the knee must remain on the floor. For an added stretch to the lateral vastus (quadriceps) muscle, bend and cross the left lower leg over the right thigh, and allow the weight of this leg to draw the right leg into increased inward rotation. Roll away from the folded leg (towards the left side of the body) before attempting to unfold it. Repeat on the second side.

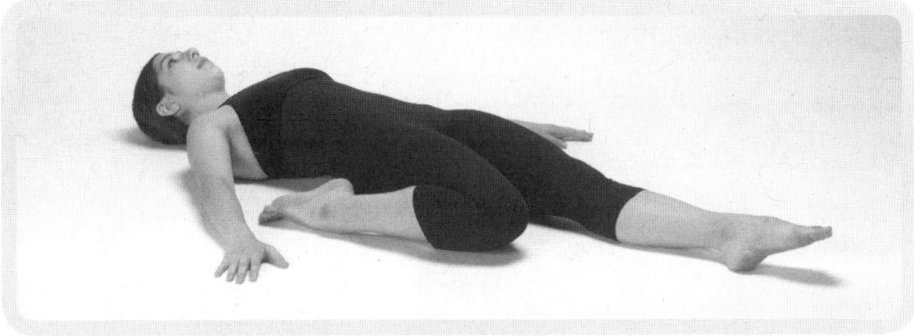

IMAGERY

For the Variation 3 – Back-Lying, imagine the lumbar spine and sacrum dropping to the floor as the pubic bone rises towards the navel. In all variations, imagine that the front of the thigh, particularly the outer thigh, is expanding and growing longer on each exhale.

7) Hip Flexor Lunge

(A) Begin by coming to all fours, supporting the weight on the knees and hands. Bring the right foot forward between the hands, and lift up into a long, low lunge with the front leg parallel, the foot under the knee (not the hips), and the back knee resting on a mat, not the hard floor. Straightening the back leg engages the rectus femoris, which would compromise the effectiveness of this stretch. The pelvis should stay as neutral as possible. The arms can be relaxed and hanging at the sides of the body or, if this too uncomfortable, the hands can remain on the floor on either side of the front foot, supporting the weight. This area of the hip can also be stretched lying supine on a bench or table, with the edge of the table or bench bisecting the two hip joints. Hold one leg at the chest to stabilize the pelvis, and allow the other leg to hang off the end of the table, imagining the hanging leg heavy and released, and the hip flexors melting and lengthening.

IMAGERY

For *Hip Flexor Lunge*, imagine that the front of the hip joint is made of soft, new taffy that stretches and yields to the weight of the torso. See the plumb line floating out of the top of the head towards the ceiling to maintain a good length in the spine. In the arching back variation (C), imagine the bottom of the rib cage floating away from the thigh as the lumbar spine lengthens. Visualize the entire neck and spine creating a huge arc, as if lying on an exercise ball.

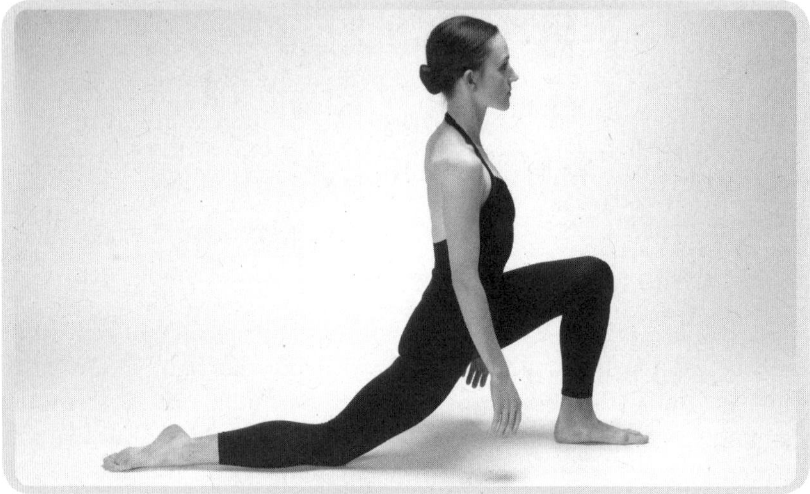

B) Bring the hands to the floor, slightly turn out the front (right) leg, and rotate the pelvis to face that leg, placing the left hand on the floor for support. Lower the left side of the pelvis towards the floor, bending the body sideways in the opposite direction (to the right). The dancer might need to move around in this position slightly until a stretch in the target area is experienced. For an added quadriceps stretch, gently fold the left knee and take hold of the left ankle with the right hand. Note: If the weight is resting directly on the knee, or if this is painful to the knee, do not attempt this variation!

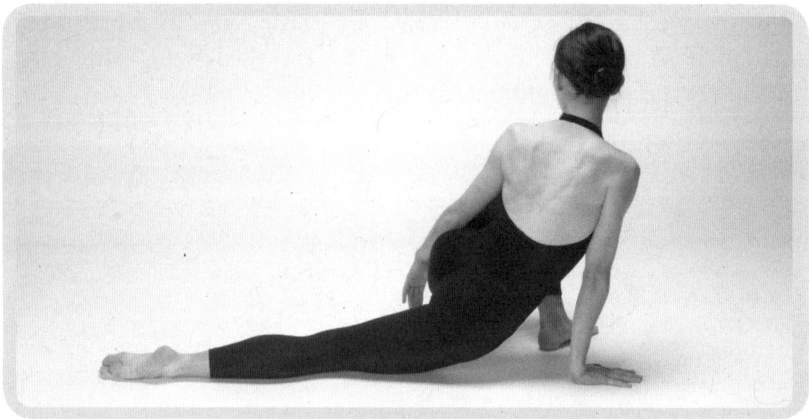

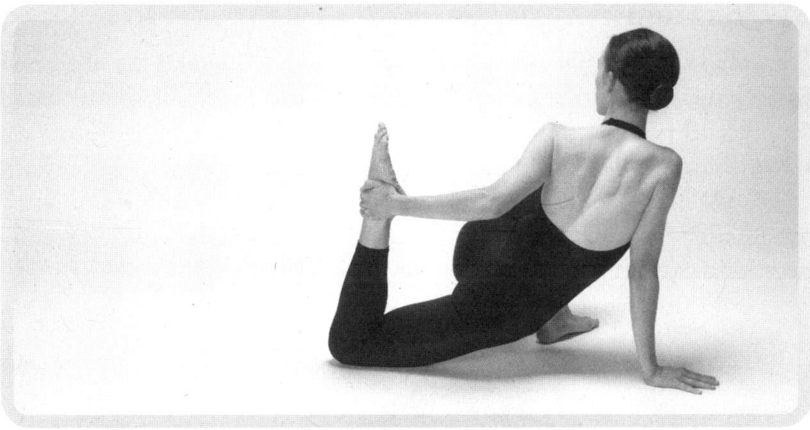

(C) Release the left foot back down to the floor, and return to the centred lunge, bringing the front leg and foot back to parallel. Place the hands on the right thigh, and while gently pressing the thigh away from the body lift the focus to the ceiling and move the rib cage up and away from the pelvis, increasing the distance between the upper thigh and the lower thoracic vertebrae. The neck should remain long and easeful. Repeat the selected version(s) on the second side.

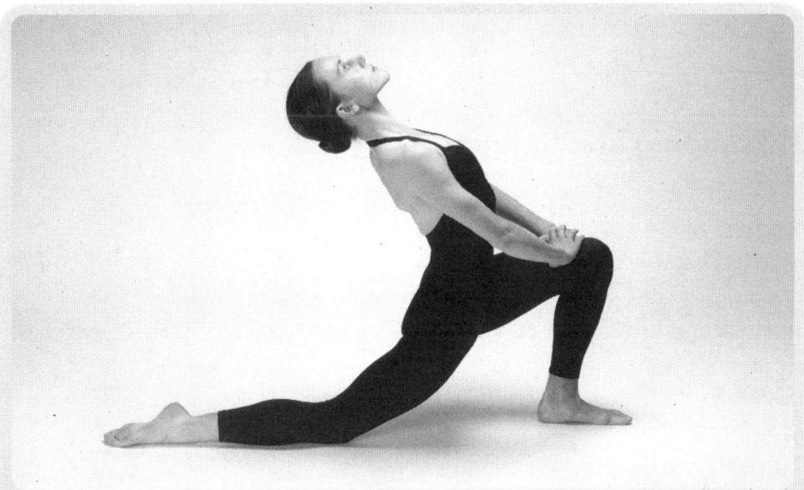

8) Mountain

Return to all fours, flex the feet, curl the toes under, and lift the hips up to the ceiling to extend both legs. The heels should be slightly off the floor in a parallel position the width of the hip sockets. If the heels are way up off of the floor, or resting flat on the floor, adjust the distance between the hands and feet until a calf stretch is experienced. Relax the neck and let the head hang. The dancer can shift from one foot to the other for an additional stretch.

IMAGERY

For *Mountain*, imagine the hands and feet spreading into the ground like roots, and the heels sinking back away from the calves. Allow the head to hang, so that a skier coming down the mountain would have one smooth path.

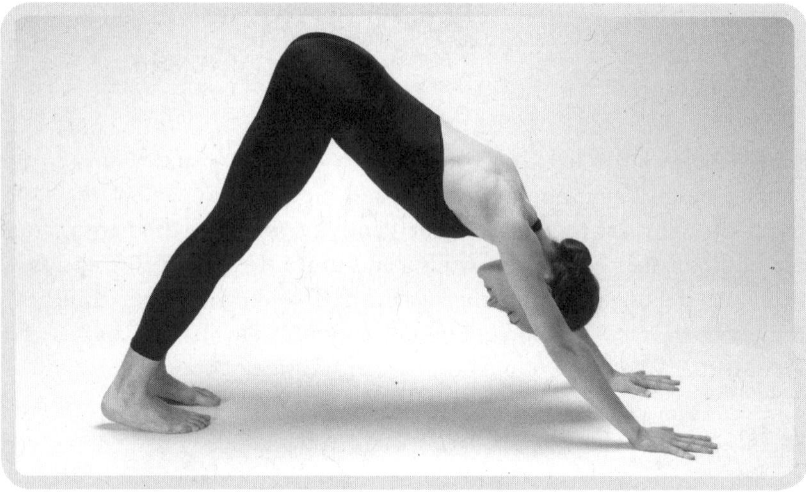

9) Standing and Hanging

(A) Walk the hands towards the feet as the knees bend. Once again, lift the hips up to the ceiling to elongate the legs for a standing hamstring stretch, keeping the weight in the centre of the feet. (B) Softly bend the knees again, and interlock the fingers behind the low back. On the exhale, again lift the hips to the ceiling to extend the legs, as the arms are lifted in a posterior direction as far as possible (i.e., in the direction of the back of the head), to stretch the front of the shoulders. Release the arms back to hanging at the end.

IMAGERY

For *Standing and Hanging*, visualize the pelvis sinking towards the front of the thighs, as the head and upper torso become heavier. The backs of the legs can be like taffy, or imagine hot water pouring down the legs.

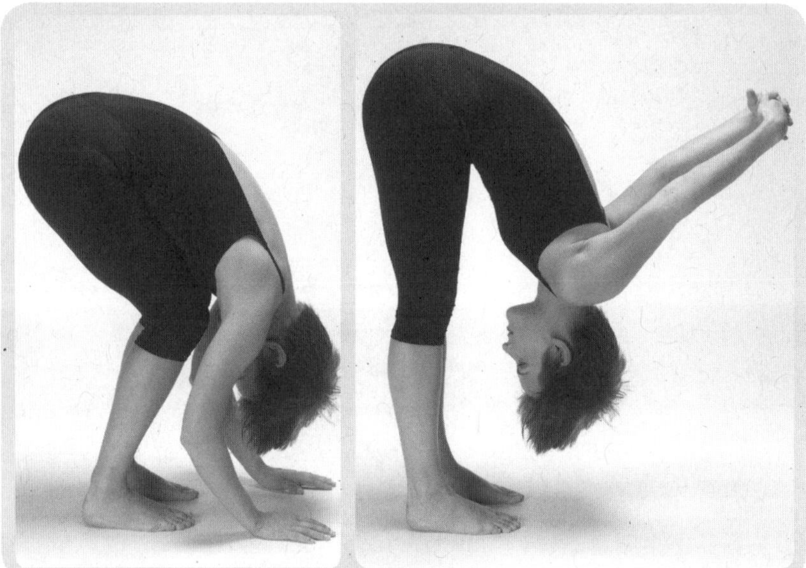

Applications and Transfer to Standing and Travelling Work

The Flexibility Series transfers to standing and travelling work by teaching dancers à mechanism for using breath and imagery to release neuromuscular tension, thereby increasing range of motion in dynamic movement. Even if dancers have considerably passive flexibility, if they have tension patterns once they begin working in stance and moving through space, they will not be able to access this full range of motion.

Notes for Teachers

Continue to remind the dancers about their breathing. Suggest ideas that encourage relaxation, and avoid force and pain. If the dancers are in pain or if the limbs begin shaking, they should back off, or modify the position until they can find a variation that is easeful.

In *Sitting with Folded Legs on a Diagonal*, make sure that the downstage shoulder is dropping towards the floor so that the dancer is in a diagonal curve and not a side bend. Additionally, tighter dancers can place the hand on the thigh they are twisting away from, and gently press it open to the floor. This additional pressure will help increase range of motion in that hip.

In *Sitting with the Soles of the Feet Together*, the feet should be placed only as close to the body as the dancer can sustain and still reach the pelvis forward of the line of gravity. Thus, for tighter dancers, the diamond should be larger.

For *Hanging over Extended Legs* and *Sitting in Second Position*, dancers who cannot comfortably sit with the pelvis forward in relation to the plumb line should do lying-down variations instead. For *Hanging over Extended Legs*, when the feet are flexed, the spine should remain long (not curved), as it can create too much tension on the sciatic nerve. In the forward-hanging versions, keep the feet relaxed, not flexed. For *Sitting in Second Position*, in side-bending, make sure the dancers keep the focus forward, not down, and the head, arm, and spine are directly to the side of the pelvis, not diagonally in front or back. Also, check that the dancers do not let the legs roll in, as this can put stress on the medial knee.

For *Quadriceps Variations*, if none of the variations on the floor are comfortable, the dancers can go to the barre or a chair, hold on for balance, and stretch the quadriceps by folding one leg and drawing the foot up to the buttock with the hand. Make sure that they keep the knee in alignment with the hip, that is, not drifting out to the side.

In *Hip Flexor Lunge*, watch for dancers who place the front foot under the pelvis instead of the front knee, which causes too much knee flexion, and compression in the joint. It is not advisable to do this stretch without a mat or pad, as it can irritate the back knee. Remind the dancers to hollow and narrow in this stretch to support the low back, and to maintain neutral pelvis as much as possible.

In *Mountain*, check that the dancers are in a parallel that is in line with the hip sockets, and that the heels are not way up off the floor. Also, check for excess neck tension.

In *Standing and Hanging*, remind the dancers to keep the weight in the centre of the foot, and not sink into the heels and backs of the knees. For less flexible dancers, the knees can remain slightly bent. Do not do variation B if this causes shoulder pain or sensations of excess movement in the joint.

PART FOUR DÉVELOPPÉ AND ROND DE JAMBE SERIES

4

Opening Remarks

The Développé Series takes material commonly done by standing dancers in technique classes and allows them to execute this material while lying on the back. In this configuration, gravity is assisting rather than fighting the weight of the legs, and the dancer can sense the organization of the spine with feedback from the floor, particularly in establishing and maintaining neutral alignment in the lumbar spine and pelvis. If the pelvis is twisting, tilting, or tucking under, there is immediate feedback from the floor, indicating that these accommodations are occurring. *Développé with Simple Rond de Jambe*, *Développé with Longer Rond de Jambe*, and *Développé with Full Rond de Jambe* add complexity in both rhythm and coordination, and demand a higher level of core support and pelvic stabilization to achieve. Some of the vocabulary used in this section, such as "creasing deeply in the socket" and "inserting the femur" is to encourage the easy glide of the femoral head in the socket, and to reduce the tension that inhibits range of motion for leg extensions. The action of "inserting the femur" for développé a la seconde (leg extensions to the side) is the same movement as that which occurs in the hip socket during the "uppies" in the *Jiggles* (see page 67), but with a slow, sustained dynamic. This terminology suggests that the femoral head rolls towards the lower (inferior) lip of the hip socket to initiate the action of the long bone of the femur extending up and out to the side for developpé. This image can assist in reducing gripping in the superficial hip flexors at the start of développés, which can actually limit range of motion.

Purpose

The main purpose of this entire series, as stated above, is to establish core support and efficient hip joint function for développés and rond de jambes. The images explored during the movements can be used in stance and travelling material as well, thereby encouraging similar muscle organization. Additionally, this series allows dancers to experience difficult and strenuous movements in a fairly relaxed state, giving them the opportunity to become aware of unnecessary tension in areas such as the neck, shoulders, and arms. By learning how to execute these dance movements with appropriate levels of tension and release, and with the pelvis in neutral alignment, dancers can potentially avoid certain injuries, such as medial snapping hip and tendonitis in the hip muscles.

1) Développé Front and Side (5-3s)

Begin lying on the back in parallel neutral stance. Keeping the legs parallel, slide the feet out along the floor, sending energy out of the top of the head and the feet. Rotate the legs out and flex the feet, maintaining the heel connection. While narrowing, draw the legs into grand plié and wrap the hands at the waist, just above the iliac crest of the pelvis on each side, or place the hands on the floor near the hips. Point the right foot, and bring it to the top of the left ankle bone. Développé the right leg to the forward high position (towards the ceiling, to the height one can sustain with the pelvis staying neutral) 1,2,3; return the right foot to the left ankle 2,2,3; développé the right leg to the side high position 3,2,3; return the right foot to the left ankle 4,2,3. Transition: Flex the right foot 5; place it down into the grand plié position 2; and point and prepare the left foot at the right ankle 3. Repeat the whole sequence with the left leg. When doing this version only, do the sequence right, left, right, left.

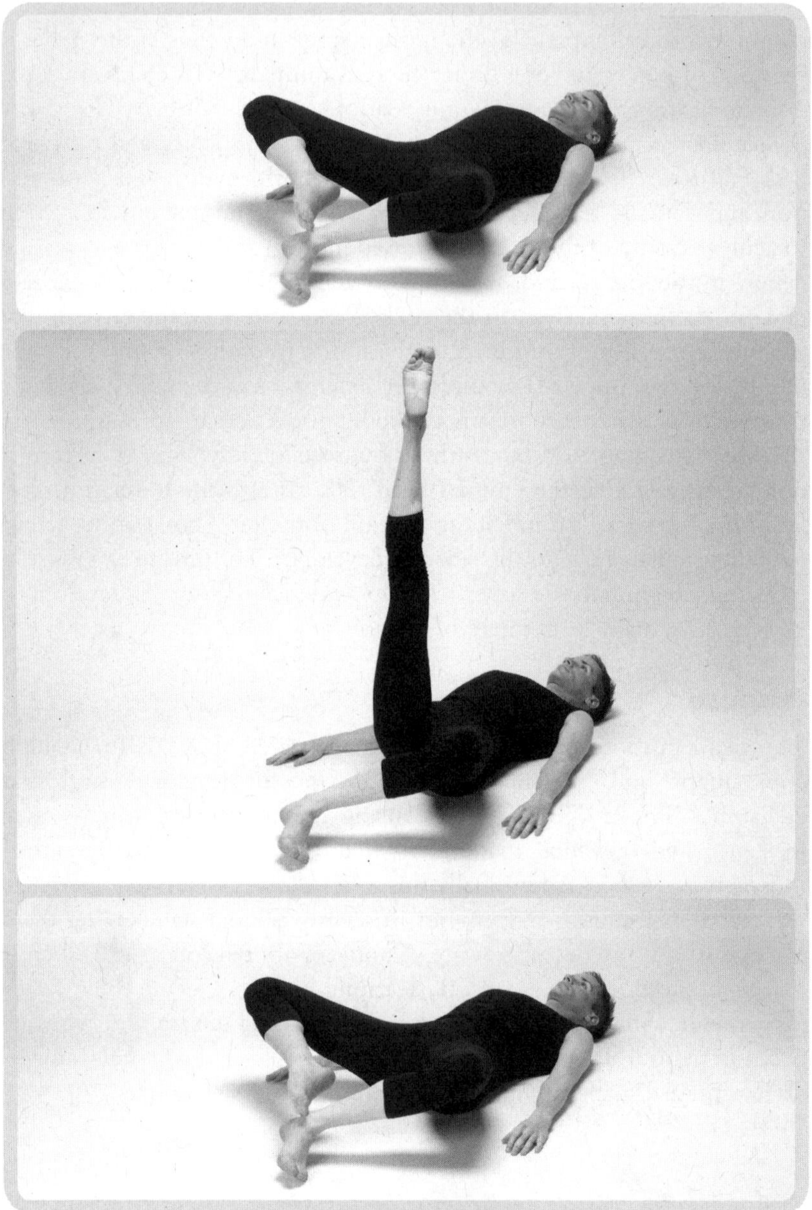

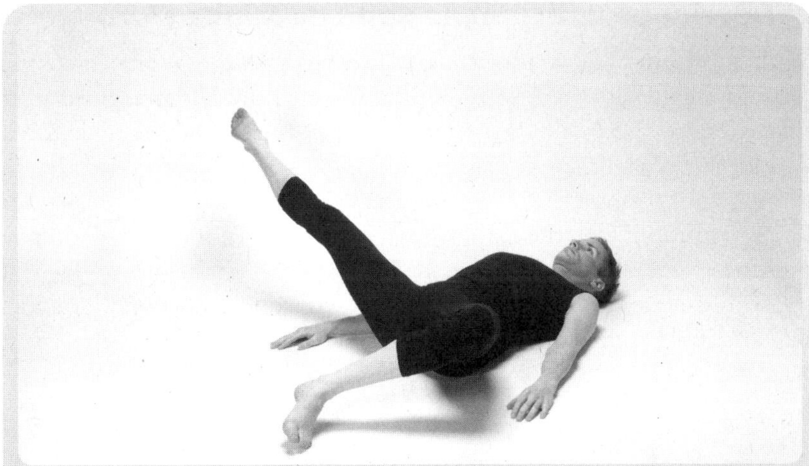

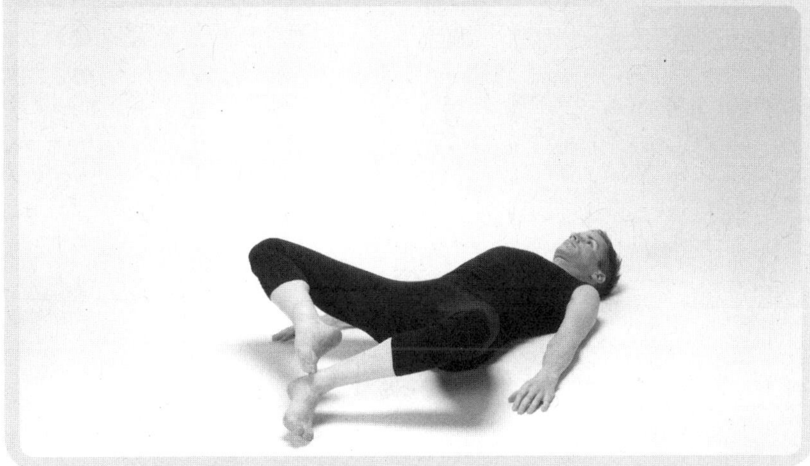

IMAGERY

For *Développé Front and Side*, imagine that the pelvis is a sandbag. Sand can pour into any part of the pelvis, giving weight to that area and maintaining neutral alignment. When extending the right leg to the front high position, all of the sand pours into the right hip to keep that side of the pelvis on the floor. As the foot returns to the ankle, the sand spreads evenly again throughout the pelvis. When extending the right leg to the side développé, all of the sand pours into the left hip, so that the pelvis does not rotate towards the extending leg, causing the left side of the pelvis to lift off the floor. Throughout the series, imagine the supporting leg actively opening wide. Imagine the extending leg as light and long, sending energy out of the foot into the distant space and continually rotating externally, as an activity and not a position. Each time the gesture leg returns to the ankle of the supporting leg, imagine both thighs widening and spreading out to the sides of the space, knees reaching to the side walls of the room. For the leg action to the front, imagine the hip socket folding and creasing deeply, with the femoral head rolling down towards the floor as the height of the leg increases. The initiation of this movement is the same action as small attitude lifts, in *Legwork in the Diamond* (see page 39). For the leg action to the side, imagine "inserting the femur" to initiate the action, seeing the femoral head gliding downward towards the heel of the supporting foot, and then unfolding the lower leg to complete the action. After the initiation (little attitude lift or inserting the femur), the awareness moves to the reach of the foot into space to emphasize the spatial intention of développé.

2) Développé with Simple Rond de Jambe (7-3s)

With the right foot at the left ankle, développé the right leg to the forward high position 1,2,3; rond de jambe the right leg, arcing to a high side extension 2,2,3; and then return the right foot to the left ankle 3,2,3; développé the right leg to the side 4,2,3; rond de jambe the right leg to the forward position 5,2,3; and return the right foot to the left ankle 6,2,3. Transition: Flex the right foot 7; place it down into the grand plié position 2; and point and prepare the left foot at the right ankle 3. Repeat the whole sequence with the left leg. When starting this second variation, do variation 1 right, left, right, left, and then variation 2, right, left. Later, a second set of variation 2 can be added, if desired.

IMAGERY

For *Développé with Simple Rond de Jambe*, dancers can continue to use the images described on page 87. Additionally, as the leg moves from front high to side on 2,2,3, imagine that both legs are doing the rond de jambe, so that the supporting leg is as energized as the gesture leg. As the leg moves from side to front high on 5,2,3, imagine the leg coiling and spiraling like a corkscrew, with the inner thigh coming around towards the chest to activate increased turnout.

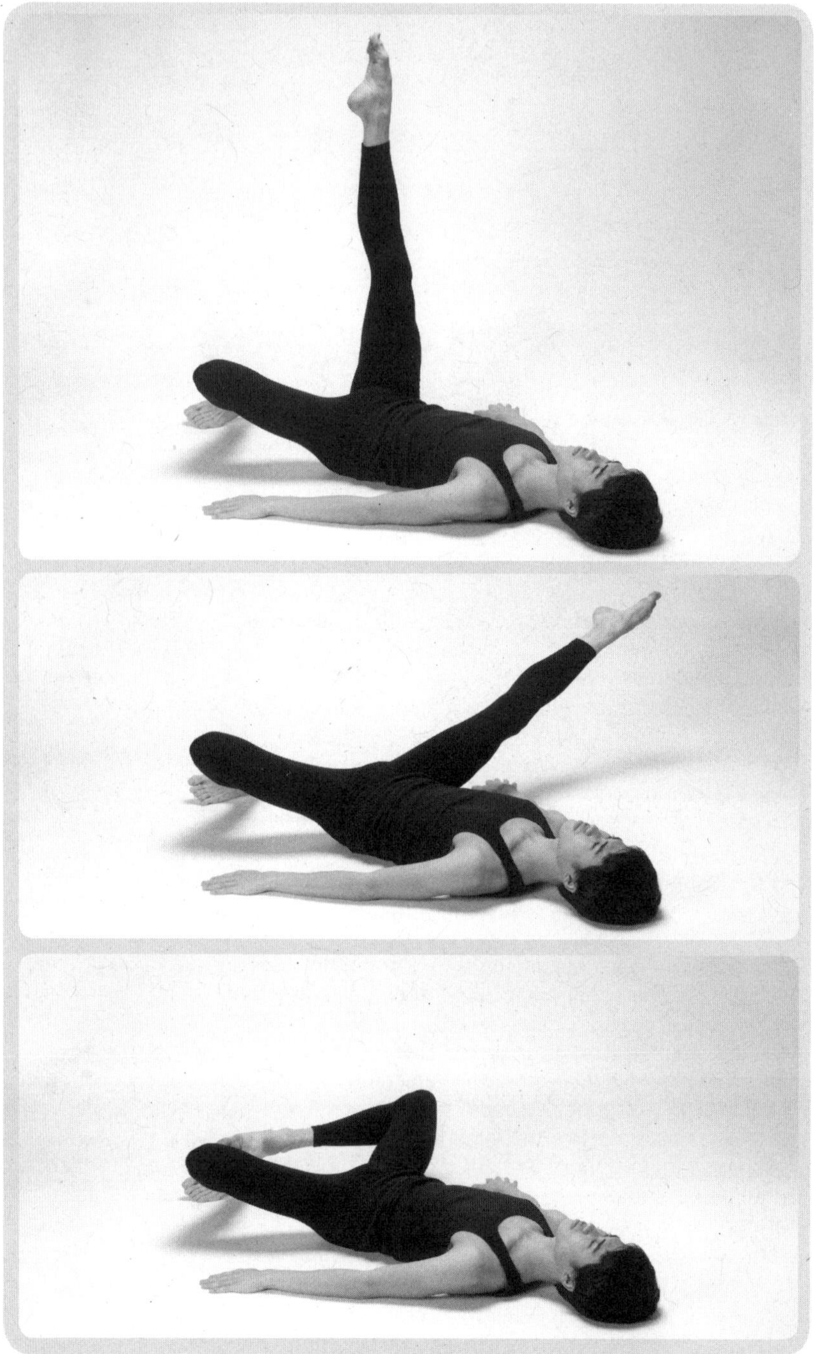

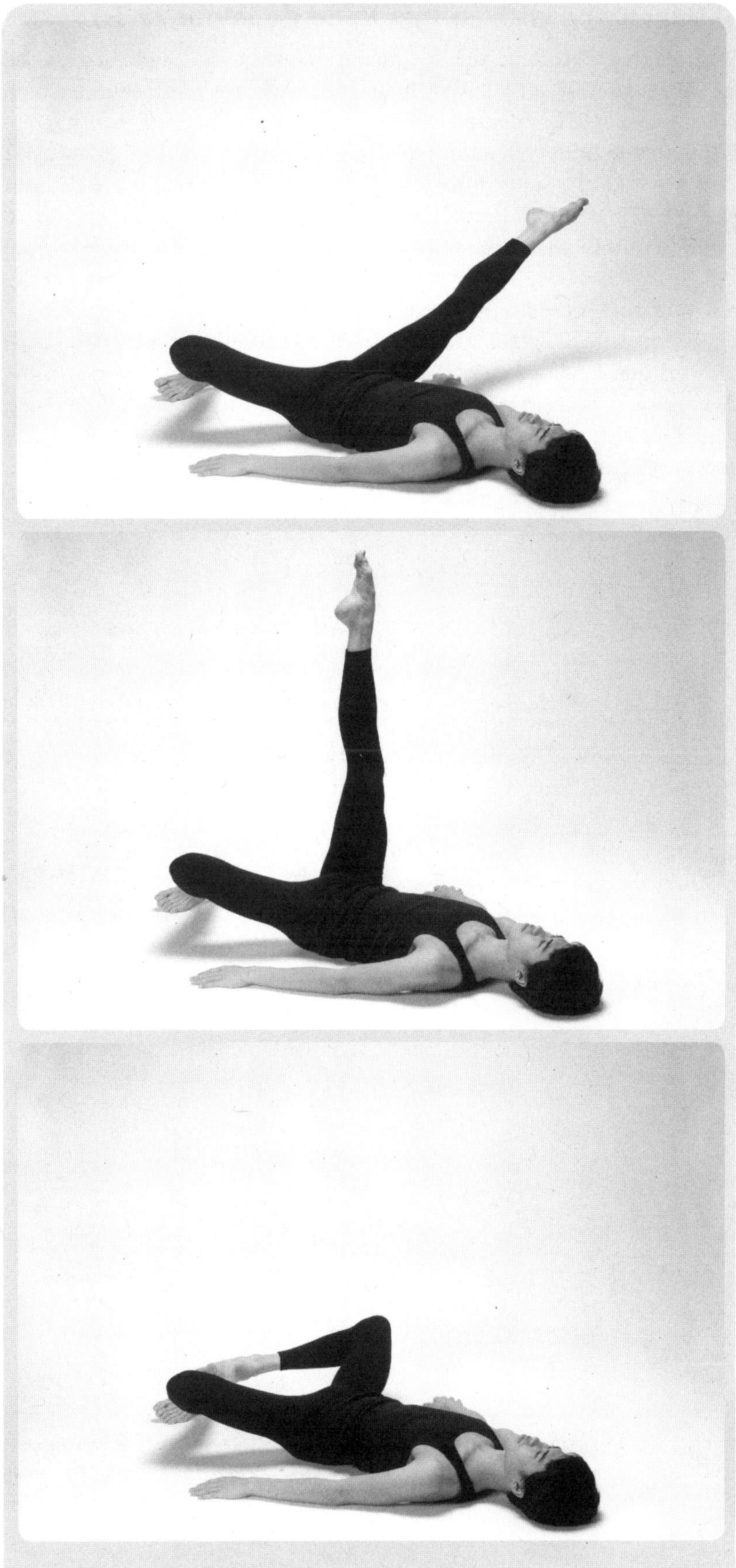

3) Développé with Longer Rond de Jambe (9-3s)

With the right foot at the left ankle, développé the right leg to the forward high position 1,2,3; rond de jambe the right leg, arcing to a high side extension 2,2,3; keeping the leg straight, reach the leg in a large arc from the side to directly under the hip joint just off the floor (that is, just to the side of the supporting left heel) 3,2,3; and return the right foot to the left ankle 4,2,3; développé the right leg to the side 5,2,3; rond de jambe the right leg to the forward high position 6,2,3; keeping the leg straight, reach the leg in a large arc from front high to directly under the hip joint just off the floor (same place as 3,2,3) 7,2,3; and return the right foot to the left ankle 8,2,3. Transition: Flex the right foot 9; place it down into the grand plié position 2; and point and prepare the left foot at the right ankle 3. Repeat the whole sequence with the left leg. When doing variations 1, 2, and 3, do variation 1 right, left, then variation 2 right, left, and then variation 3 right, left.

IMAGERY

For *Développé with Longer Rond de Jambe*, as the leg goes from the side extension to the position underneath the hip on 3,2,3, imagine the torso on the supporting leg side elongating as the leg moves downward and, at the same time, imagine the hip of the gesture leg softening like taffy and releasing to allow the leg to move freely. The image of the extending leg as light and long, sending energy out of the foot into the distant space, will assist in the releasing action of the hip muscles. As the leg moves from front high to the position underneath the hip on 7,2,3, imagine an increase of the narrowing and hollowing as the leg lowers, seeing an oppositional line of energy up the front of the body from the pubic bone to the navel. As the leg lowers, one can also imagine the taffy in the front of the hip joint softening and elongating.

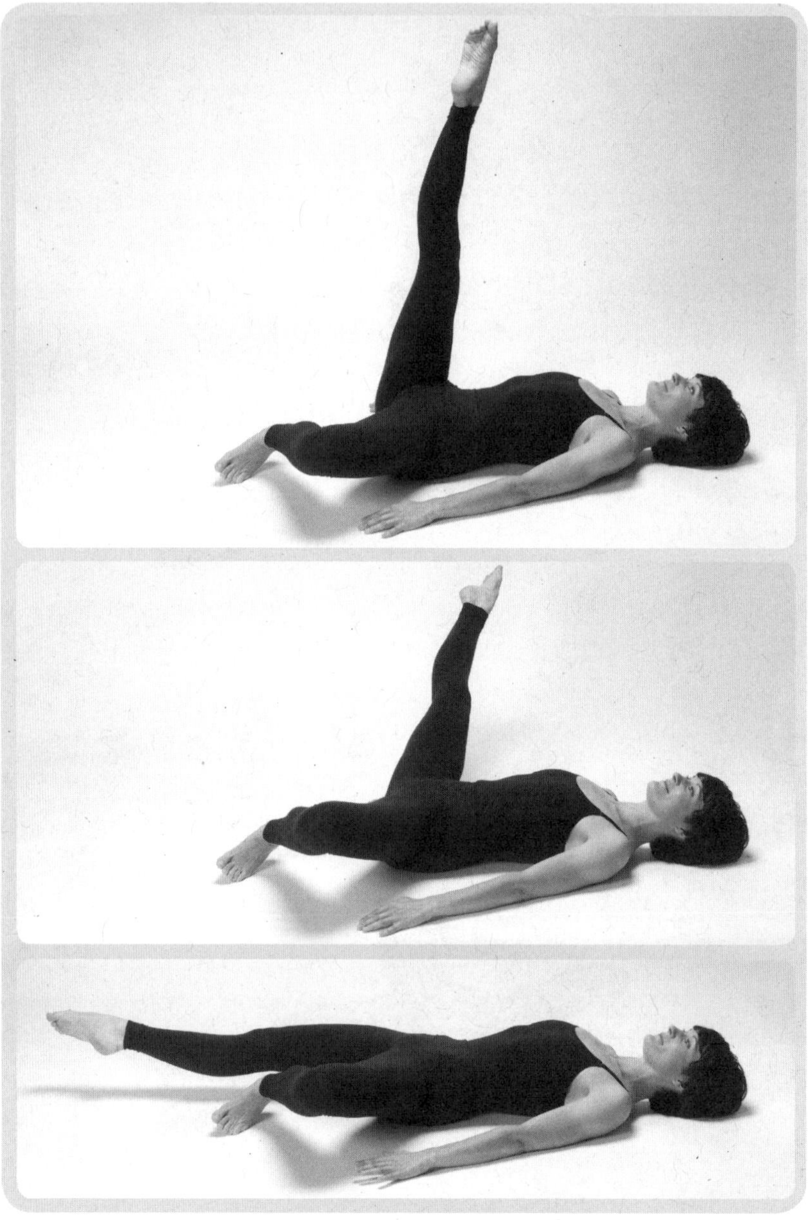

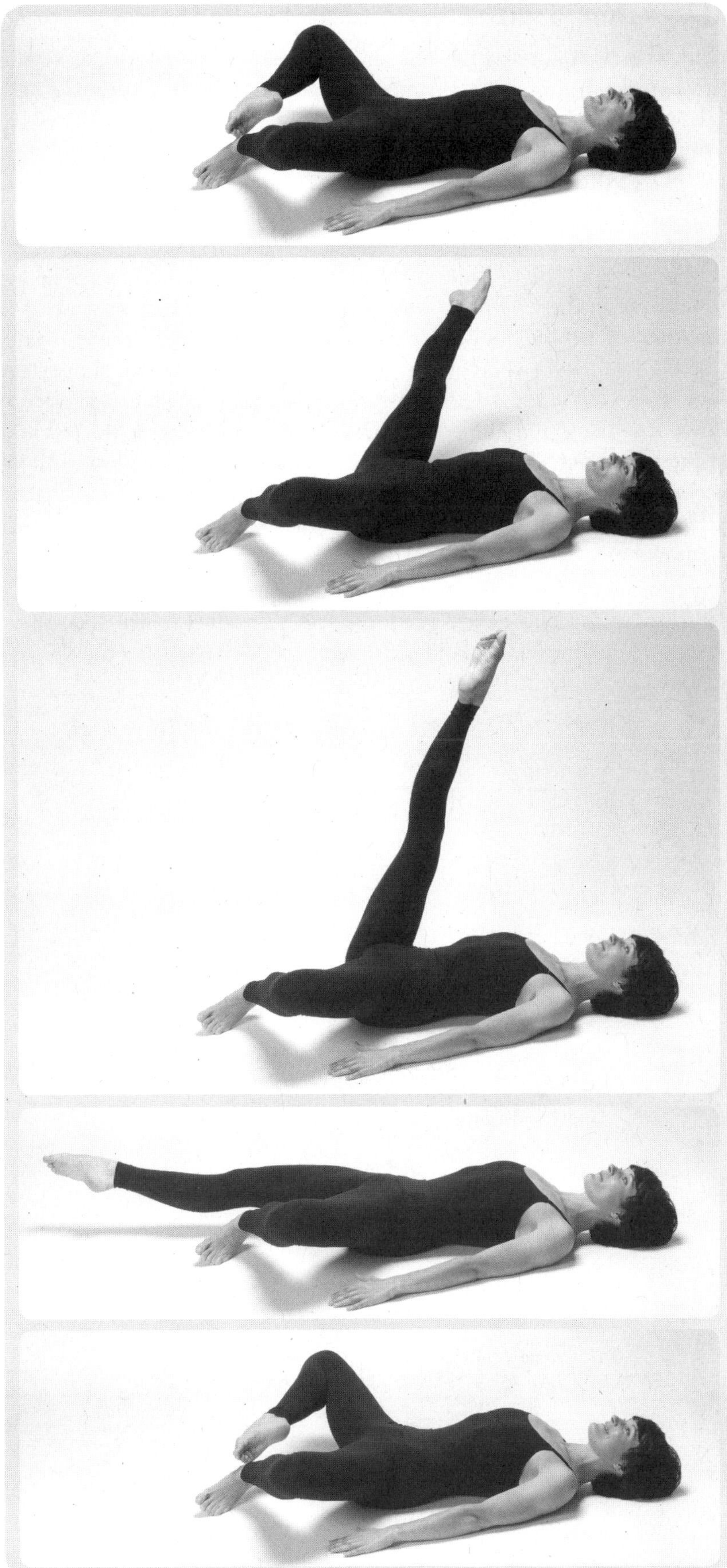

4) Développé with Full Rond de Jambe (11-3s)

With the right foot at the left ankle, développé the right leg to the forward high position 1,2,3; rond de jambe the right leg, arcing to a high side extension 2,2,3; keeping the leg straight, reach the leg in a large arc from side to directly under the hip joint just off the floor (that is, just to the side of the supporting left heel) 3,2,3; reach the leg up to the front high position (where it was on 1,2,3) on 4,2,3; and return the right foot to the left ankle 5,2,3; développé the right leg to the side 6,2,3; rond de jambe the right leg to the forward high position 7,2,3; keeping the leg straight, reach the leg in a large arc from front high to directly under the hip joint just off the floor (same place as 3,2,3) 8,2,3; reach the leg to the side high position (where it was on 6,2,3) on 9,2,3; and return the right foot to the left ankle 10,2,3. Transition: Flex the right foot 11; place it down into the grand plié position 2; and point and prepare the left foot at the right ankle 3. Repeat the whole sequence with the left leg. This variation completes the full circle from the starting extension to the final position before returning to the ankle. For all the variations, do one set right and one set left.

At the end of the series (no matter which variation is the final version), return to grand plié, gently bring the legs to parallel stance, slide them out along the floor, and take some time to rest, easily shaking out the legs and rocking them in and out.

IMAGERY

For *Développé with Full Rond de Jambe*, as the leg moves from the low position underneath the hip to front high on 4,2,3, imagine the glue on the back of the sacrum getting stronger and the hip socket deeply creasing and folding. As the leg moves from the low position underneath the hip to side high on 9,2,3, imagine the torso on the gesture leg side elongating as the leg moves upward, while the iliac crest on the supporting side stays connected to the bottom of the rib cage. In both directions, remember to keep the energy pouring out of the foot and into distant space, and the corkscrew image alive.

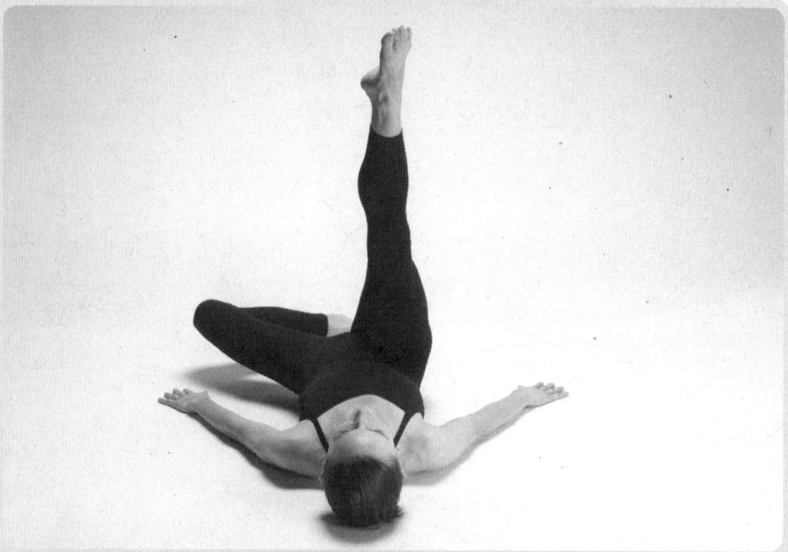

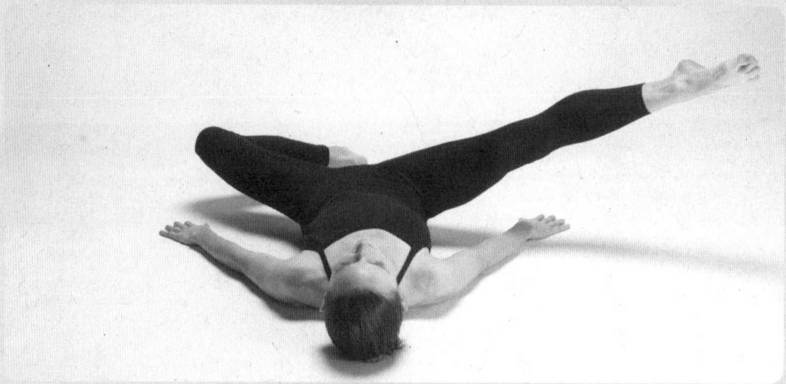

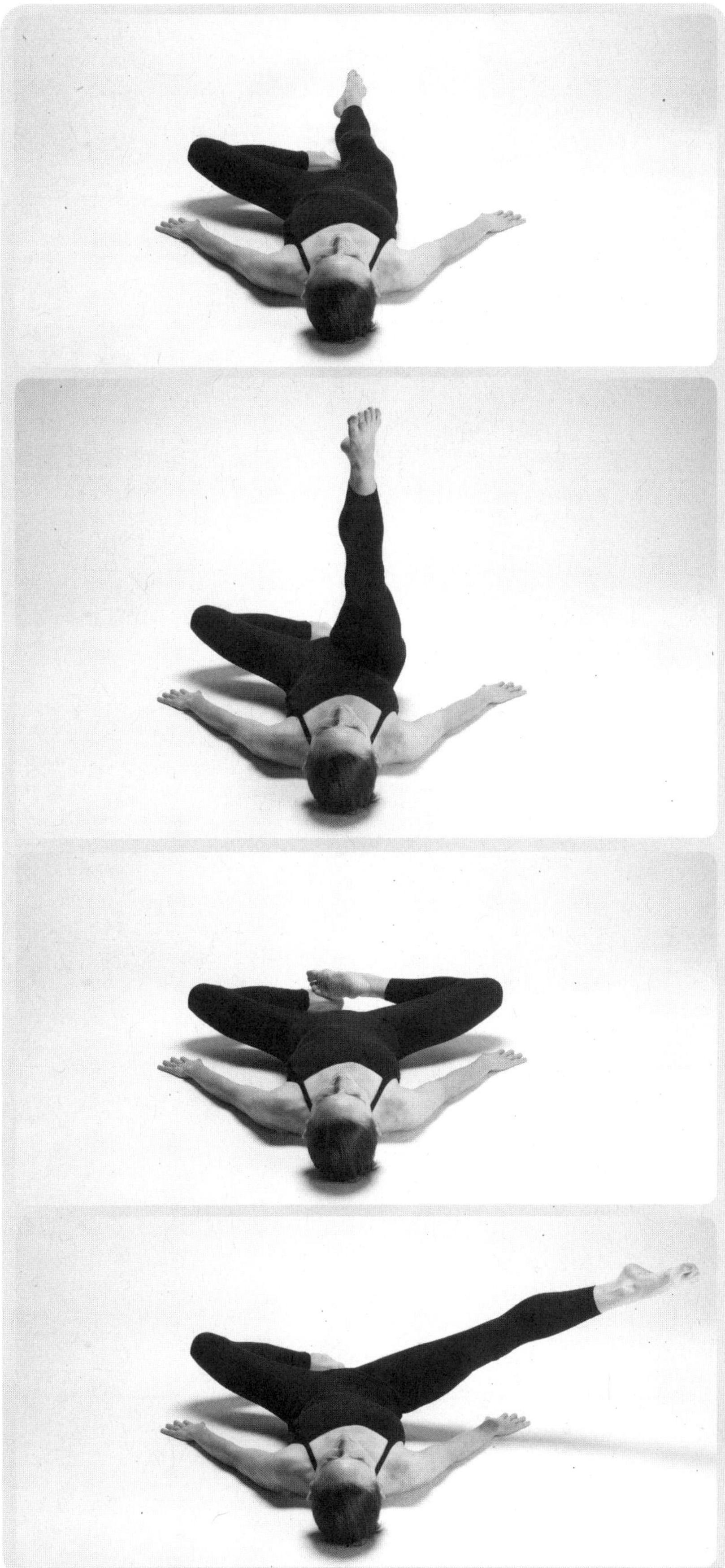

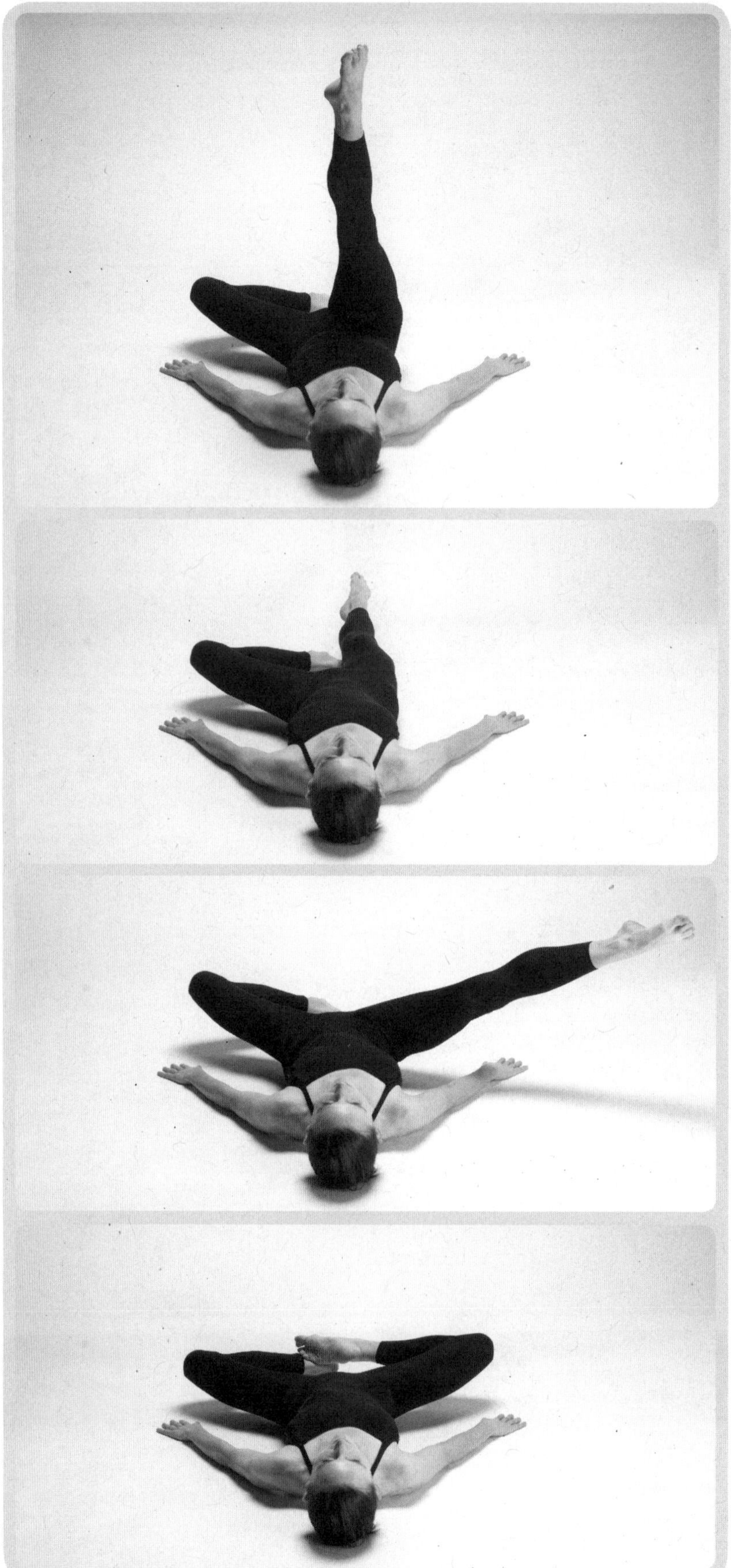

Notes for Teachers

The use of the legs in grand plié, rather than an extended supporting leg, for this series, provides counterbalance to the weight of the gesture leg. When dancers are first starting the développés, they can place the arms on the floor at shoulder height (palms down), and then by the hips to support some of the weight. As they become more advanced, dancers can place the arms in second position off the floor, and finally in fifth position. Each of these variations increases the challenge to the core of the body.

Make sure that the dancers are narrowing and hollowing throughout, and see that they avoid bracing the surface abdominals and tucking under in the pelvis, especially at the start of the series and as the gesture leg returns to the supporting ankle each time. Both of these deviations will create excessive tension, especially to the psoas, and stress on its tendon, and possibly impede breathing. To avoid tucking, encourage the use of the image of the sacrum glued to the floor, and the tailbone reaching to connect to the floor.

It is important not to progress through the variations too quickly. If the dancers feel cracking and snapping in the hips, the first strategy to attempt is to deepen the narrowing and hollowing. Also, encourage use of the images of reaching the leg away from the pelvis into space, and seeing the surface muscles softening and elongating. If the snapping persists, try reducing the range of motion, and if nothing seems to achieve a smooth action, it may mean the dancers should return to a simpler variation. They may need more hip flexor (including iliopsoas) stretching, and adductor strengthening, or more active recruitment of core muscles. For younger dancers, it may also be the case that they are going through a growth spurt and need to limit the range of motion substantially, or even forego développés for a brief period.

Be aware of the dancer's rib cage placement and movement. Ribs pushing up off the floor can indicate excess tension in the muscles of the spine in the thoracic area. Rib tension can also suggest a lack of good breathing rhythm. For dancers who have excessive tension in the legs and hips, it is useful to exhale on the extension phase. For dancers who tend to compress the spine in stance, it is useful to inhale on the extension phase. Most importantly, breathe!

The bottom foot (support leg) should stay in full dorsiflexion and that leg should maintain its external rotation with the hamstrings fairly relaxed. Remember to emphasize that the height of the gesture leg is less important than maintaining neutral pelvis and core support.

PART FIVE DEVELOPING TURNOUT

Opening Remarks

This section is executed lying on the side of the body. There are four goals:

(1) To develop the strength, trunk support, and awareness for proper use of turnout in dance

(2) To challenge the core and the balance of the body on a narrow base of support, relative to lying on the back

(3) To encourage muscle balance in the various muscle groups that surround the hip joint

(4 To promote range of motion in the hips for dance aesthetics

It is crucial that the dancer be sufficiently advanced, both physically and in terms of body awareness, to maintain the alignment of the trunk, and the arm and leg that are on the floor throughout the series.

A – Clams

Purpose

Because gravity is in a different relationship to the body when side-lying, this series is a far greater challenge in terms of working on turnout with the necessary core support. Therefore, the integration of core support and external rotation can be emphasized. Additionally, gravity is no longer assisting in maintaining neutral alignment (head, rib cage, and pelvis) adding challenge to the musculature and motor patterning for achieving this organization.

Learning that the placement of the gesture leg in passé is slightly anterior to the pelvis is crucial for the health of the standing knee. When the dancer forces the passé too far back, it rotates the pelvis in that direction, putting torque on the standing knee, as the foot remains in the same position on the floor. This torque gradually stresses the knee ligaments, and can create instability in the knee joint.

This series also focuses on continued work recruiting the deep external rotators of the hip, and not relying exclusively on the gluteus maximus for turnout. This use of the deep muscles diminishes surface tension (i.e., in the superficial muscles) that can restrict range of motion and block fluidity in movement quality.

1) Baby Clam

The *Baby Clam* is a preparation for the *Full Clam*. Begin lying on the back, in parallel neutral stance. Bring the arms to an oval in front of the rib cage. Move the left arm to fifth position. Roll onto the left side of the body, extending the left arm along the floor directly above the torso, palm down, and resting the side of the head on the arm. The right hand is placed on the floor in front of the rib cage, supporting some of the weight if needed. The knees remain bent at 90°, feet pointed, as the legs arrive on the floor in front of the hips. The feet should now be directly under the pelvic floor. Note: The feet will adjust slightly forward during this transition, or they will end up behind the pelvis. The waist is elevated off the floor by increasing the narrowing and hollowing, and aligning the ribs and pelvis. Once this position is clearly established, the *Baby Clam* can begin: Open the right (top) thigh to a full passé, keeping the feet connected, on counts 1,2; close the thigh back down to the left thigh on 3,4. The pelvis and ribs remain quiet throughout the movement. Repeat eight times. Return to neutral parallel stance lying on the back. Repeat on the second side for the left leg.

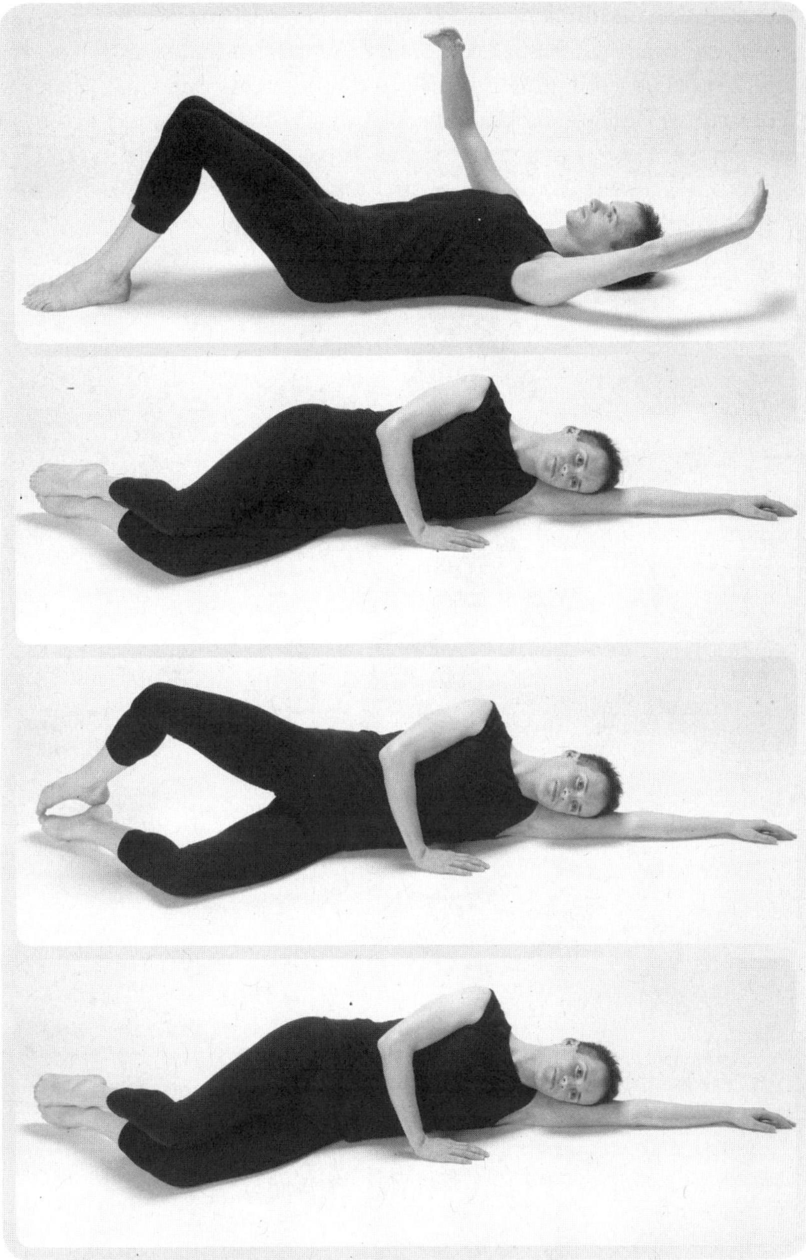

IMAGERY

For all three clam variations, imagine the body is perched on a balance beam. The top hand and arm, the rib cage, the pelvis, and the underneath foot (and entire leg in *Full Clam* and *Beyond the Clam*) are all along the balance beam. The top knee is in front of the beam in *Baby Clam*, and the front (right) hand is forward of the beam in all three variations, resting on an imaginary table.

Imagine a stiff wire hanging from the ceiling that drops down through the top (right) hip socket and continues down through the bottom (left) hip into the floor. This wire prevents the pelvis from rocking back and forth as the leg turns out and in, keeping the action isolated to the femur in the hip socket.

Imagine that a partner has a hand placed under the waist, holding it up off the floor, and that the waist continues to narrow away from this partner's hand. Imagine the partner has the other hand placed at the back of the hip, preventing the pelvis from rocking back as the leg turns out.

Visualize a line of energy from the bottom of the rib cage in front to the ASIS bones on the front of the pelvis, maintaining the organization of the ribs and pelvis throughout the series.

2) Full Clam

Begin lying on the back in parallel neutral stance. Bring the arms to an oval in front of the rib cage, while extending both legs along the floor, with pointed feet. Move the left arm to fifth position, and the right leg to parallel passé. In one clear action, roll onto the left side of the body, turning out both legs. As in *Baby Clam*, extend the left arm along the floor directly above the torso, palm down, and rest the side of the head on the arm. The right hand is placed on the floor in front of the rib cage, supporting some of the weight if needed. The right knee is now in a turned out passé, with the foot pointed and the big toe touching the inside of the left knee, and the left leg is on the floor in line with the left hip socket. Note: The left leg will adjust slightly forward during this transition, or it will end up behind the pelvis. There is one long, established line from the tips of the left fingers down to the left toes. The waist is elevated off of the floor by increasing the narrowing and hollowing, and aligning the ribs and pelvis. Once this position is clearly established, the *Full Clam* can begin: Inward rotate the right hip, bringing the thigh parallel to the floor on counts 1,2; open the right thigh to a full turned out passé, keeping the foot connected to the left knee, on 3,4. The pelvis and ribs remain quiet throughout the movement. Repeat eight times. Return to neutral parallel stance lying on the back. Repeat on the second side for the left leg.

IMAGERY

For *Full Clam* and *Beyond the Clam*, imagine that someone takes hold of the bottom foot and pulls it out along the floor away from the pelvis throughout the series. This leg should be actively reaching, not passively resting on the floor.

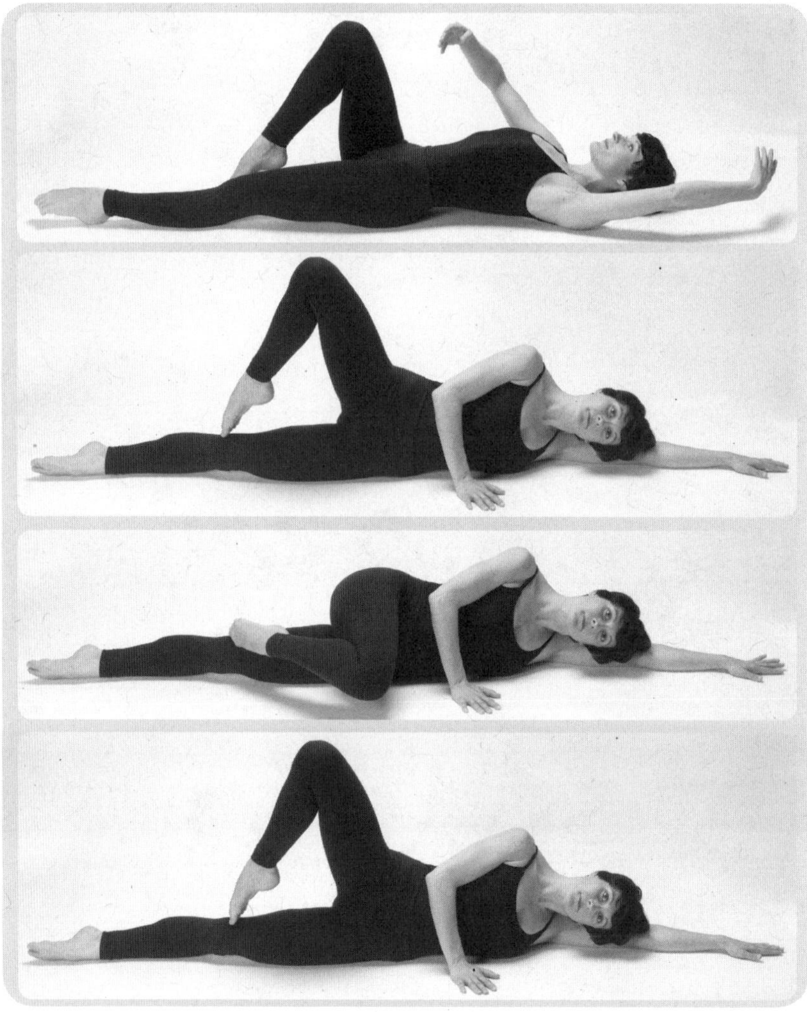

3) Beyond the Clam

Begin with the same transition onto the side of the body as in the *Full Clam*. From the turned out passé, extend the right leg to full side extension. Note: The leg will be on a slight forward diagonal, not directly to the ceiling, due to most dancers' hip structure.

Variation 1 – Rotations on a Slow 4: Flex the top foot on count 1, demi plié to a long attitude, increasing the outward rotation and height of the leg on 2, point the foot on 3, extend the leg back out to the side high position, maintaining the rotation and height on 4. Repeat four times, and do one more flex and plié to end in a side attitude.

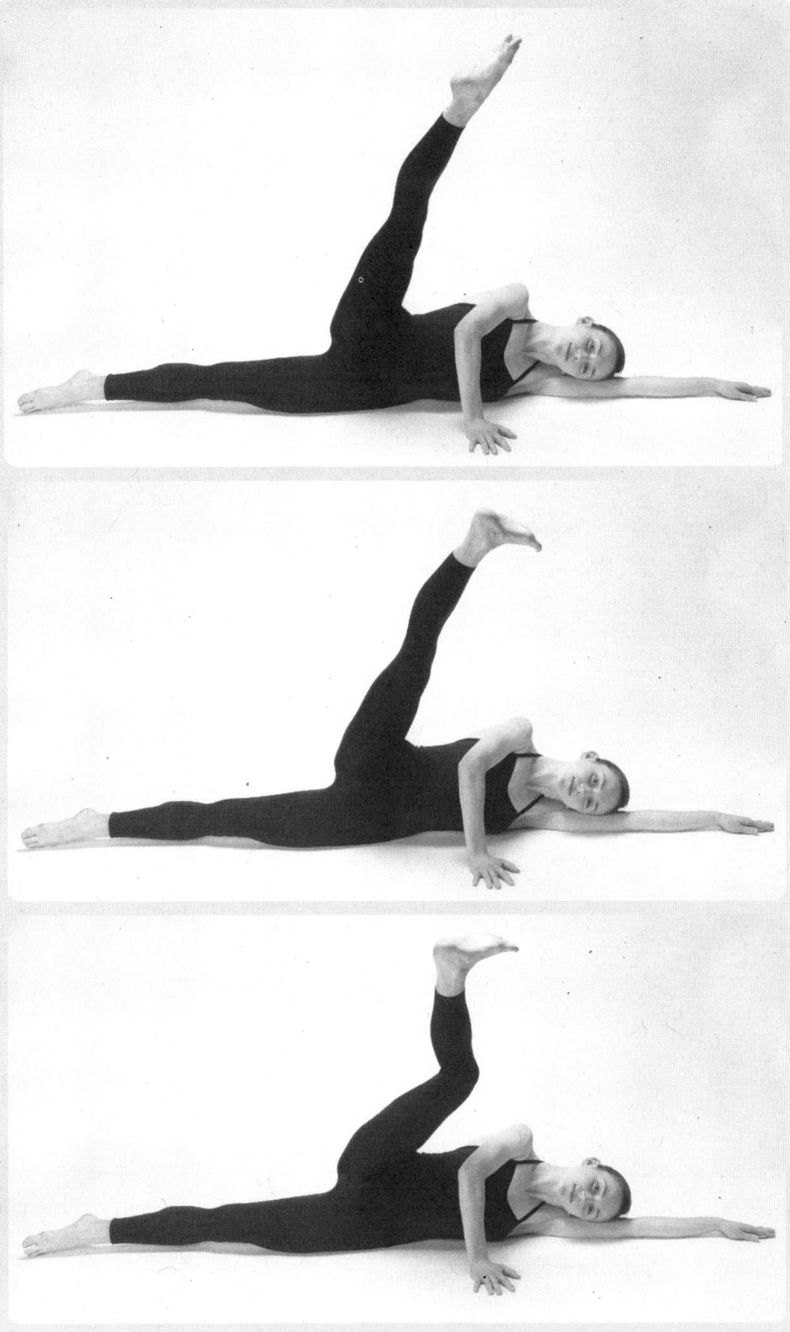

Photo Sequence continues on next page.

IMAGERY

For Variation 1 – Rotations on a Slow 4, imagine the leg as a barbershop pole as it extends out on count 4, and visualize both legs extending and rotating at the same time.

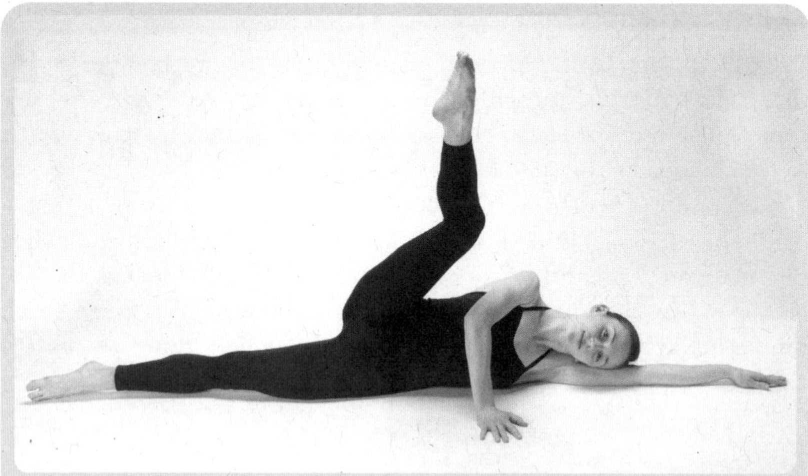

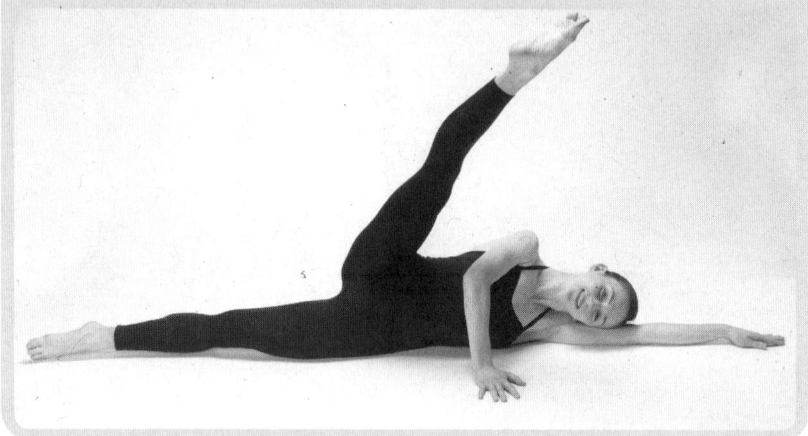

Variation 2 – Pulses on a Fast 3/8: Pulse the right leg in the hip socket in a loose action, moving the thigh in the direction of the top shoulder four times, repeat with the foot pointed four times, pulse with a flexed foot two times, with a pointed foot two times, and then alternating flex, point, flex, point for four pulses. With each pulse, focus on increasing the external rotation at the hip joint. To finish this section, extend the leg to side high once more, and fold to passé. From here, the dancers can return to neutral parallel on the back to do the second side, or proceed to the next section: A Trip Around the Hip.

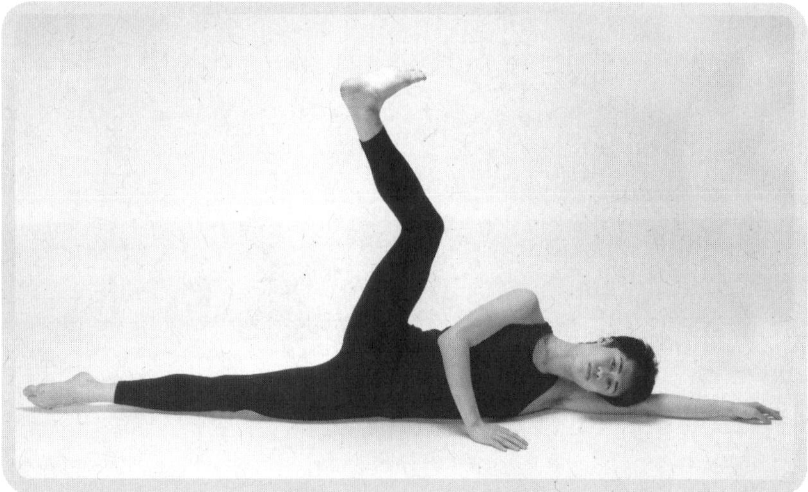

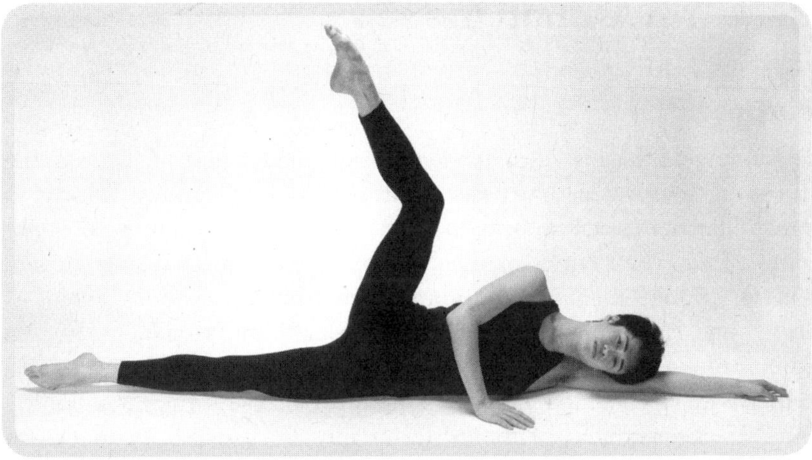

Applications and Transfer to Standing and Travelling Work

This series can be directly applied to standing work. As stated above, the clam series teaches the dancer the appropriate placement of the passé in relationship to the pelvis and standing leg, and this relationship can then be experienced when the dancer comes to stance. Additionally, the connection of core support to turnout is critical for control and ease of the use of turnout in dynamic movement on the legs. By integrating these two major concepts (core support and turnout), this series assists in transferring the use of turnout to dynamic dancing.

Notes for Teachers

One of the best ways to teach this series is to have the dancers work in pairs. One dancer gets into the side-lying position for the series, while the partner assists with hands-on work. If the dancer is lying on the left side, and the right leg is the gesture leg, the partner's left hand is placed under the waist of the dancer, and the partner's right hand is placed on the right posterior pelvis. The left hand is there to remind the dancer to stay narrowed and keep the waist off of the floor. The right hand is placed to prevent the right side of the dancer's pelvis from rocking back behind the left hip during the turnout phase of the clam. (In stance, this would be equivalent to rotating the pelvis to the right as the right leg comes to passé turned out.) Once the dancer has experienced this stabilization effort with support, it is more likely that it can be achieved without the partner's aid.

Once the pelvis is stable, the *Baby Clam* can be skipped, and the dancers can begin with the *Full Clam*. Eventually, the dancers can start side-lying work with *Beyond the Clam*.

It is best if the gesture leg does not actually touch the floor in the inward rotation phase of the *Full Clam*. While some dancers will have this range of motion, if they allow the knee to touch the floor, they tend to relax all of the muscular support for the leg, which is inappropriate for standing work.

Finally, remind the dancers to attend to the standing leg in *Full Clam* and *Beyond the Clam*. This leg should remain actively extended and turned out, with energy flowing out of the end of the pointed foot. Similarly, the upper arm should remain extended in the long "balance beam" line, and not drift forward along the floor, in conjunction with a soft rib cage.

B – A Trip Around the Hip

Purpose

Expanding on the goals described in the opening remarks of "Developing Turnout," the primary purpose of this section of side-lying work is to strengthen the lateral and medial muscles around the hip that are not emphasized when lying on the back, including the abductors/inward rotators (gluteus medius and minimus), the adductors, and the extensors (hamstrings and gluteus maximus). Additionally, this section is designed to ensure balanced use of these muscle groups. The lateral and medial muscles are essential for stability in the hip, especially when standing on one leg. Recruitment of the posterior muscles is necessary to extend the standing hip correctly, and to support leg gestures to the back (e.g., tendu, degagé, and arabesque). *Dancing Legs* encourages use of greater range of motion in the hips, while promoting core support, which may aid in preventing injury to the low back in high legwork. The *Spiral Stretch* allows a rest and recuperation phase for muscles that have just been working strenuously. Finally, the *Beats* add fast tempo and dynamic to the recruitment of the inner thigh muscles, while connecting this muscular action to core support work.

1) Leg Lifts for the Outer Leg

At the end of the *Full Clam* or *Beyond the Clam*, the dancer is side-lying with the underneath leg extended and turned out, and the gesture leg in turned out passé. Bend the underneath leg to 90° and turn it parallel, so that the thigh stays in line (on the balance beam) with the hip joint, and the foot is placed directly behind the knee. Rotate the gesture leg to parallel and flex the foot. Extend the gesture leg directly in front of the body, keeping it just off of the floor, while sending energy out of the heel. Now reach the leg in a downward arc until it is directly over the standing thigh, still parallel. Rotate the leg slightly inward (if possible) so that the toes are lower than the heel. Maintaining the space under the waist, on count 1, lift the leg side as high as possible, without moving the pelvis or allowing the leg to rotate out. Return the leg to its starting position on count 2. Do eight repetitions, finishing on the lift. (Advanced dancers continue to *Pressing to the Back*.) For intermediate dancers, do the following transition, and then go on to *Leg Lifts for the Inner Leg*. Point the foot, turn the leg out, and reach it to a back attitude, touching the toes to the floor behind the pelvis. Maintain a strong connection of the pubic bone to the navel, and the rib cage to the pelvis. Return to the passé, pelvis back to neutral.

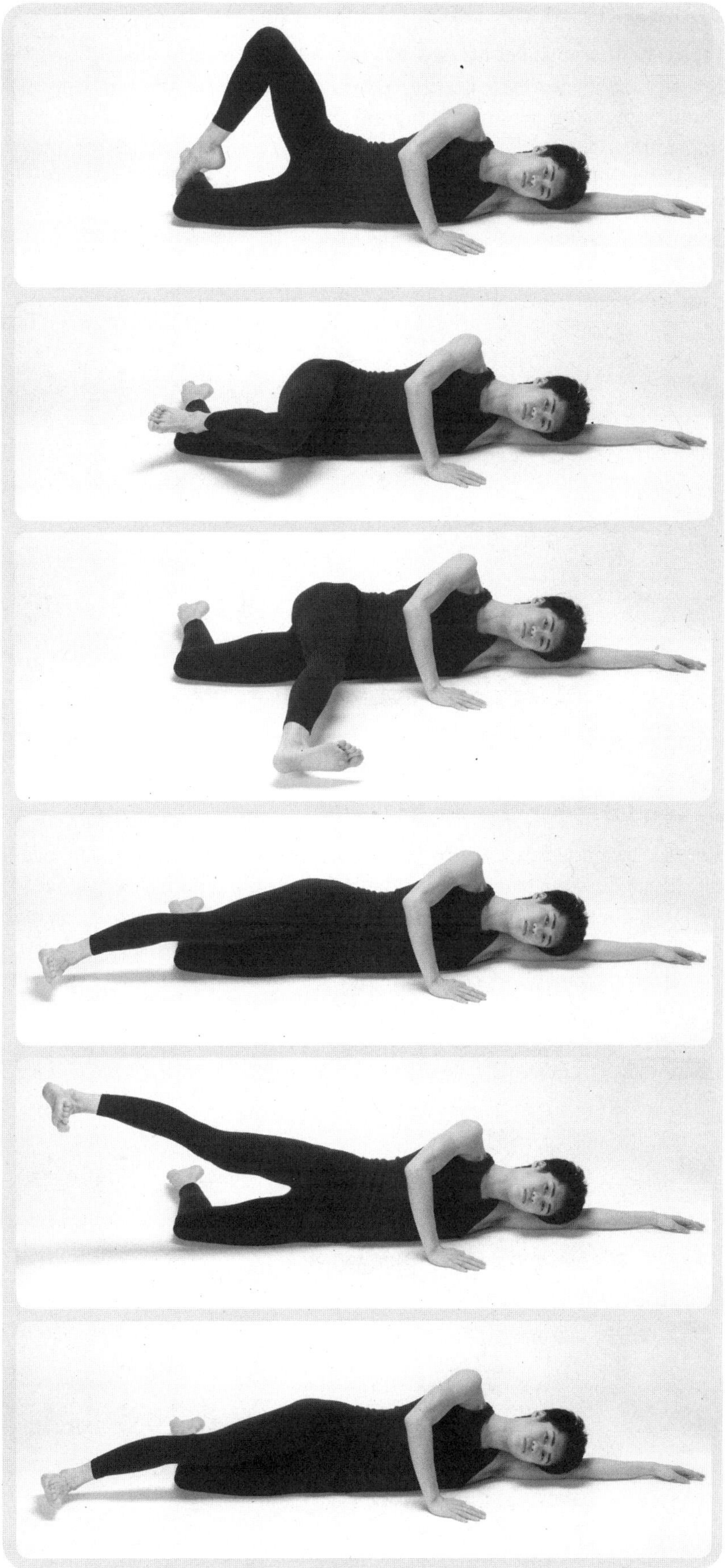

IMAGERY

For this entire sequence, continue to visualize the body perched on a balance beam, with energy flowing out of the head and toes. When the leg underneath bends, the thigh remains on the beam, while the lower leg reaches out behind the beam. Imagine the narrowing and hollowing increasing as the series progresses, and a strong line of energy connecting the rib cage and the pelvis.

For *Leg Lifts for the Outer Leg*, imagine a hand placed under the waist that maintains the space between the waist and the floor. The heel of the moving leg should be pressing out against an imaginary wall as the thigh rotates in. At the end, as the leg returns to passé from the back attitude, imagine that the pelvis moves back to neutral, and carries the leg with it to arrive under the torso.

2) Pressing to the Back

From the final parallel lift above, maintain the flexed foot, and turn the leg out. Lower it down until the foot is in line with the hip joint. On count 1, press the leg directly behind the pelvis, like a tendu to the back, maintaining the core support. On count 2, come back to neutral, with the leg in line with the hip. Do eight repetitions, finishing the last one with the leg behind the pelvis. Point the foot, turn the leg out, and reach it to a back attitude, touching the toes to the floor behind the pelvis. Maintain a strong connection of the pubic bone to the navel, and the rib cage to the pelvis. Return to the passé, pelvis back to neutral.

IMAGERY

For *Pressing to the Back*, imagine the elastics from *Undercurves and Overcurves* connecting the pubic bone to the navel. The elastics lengthen but remain taut on the press back, and draw the pubic bone forward on the return movement. As in *Leg Lifts for the Outer Leg*, the heel presses out into the space, but now the thigh rotates out continually.

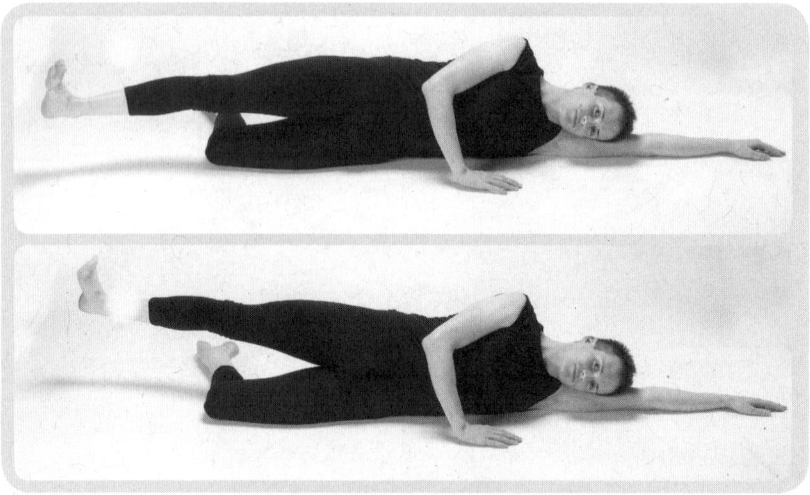

3) Leg Lifts for the Inner Leg

Extend the underneath leg and turn it out. Flex the top foot, and place it directly behind the hamstrings of the long leg on the floor, standing on the foot. On count 1, maintaining the turnout, lift the underneath leg as high off the floor as possible, keeping it in line with the hip. On count 2, return it to the floor. Do eight repetitions, finishing with the leg off the floor. Lower the bottom leg back to the floor, return to passé once again (check that the pelvis is in neutral), and slowly développé the top leg to high second position. Intermediate dancers, skip *Dancing Legs* and go on to *Spiral Stretch*.

IMAGERY

For *Leg Lifts for the Inner Leg*, visualize the lifting leg directly under the hip joint and the leg getting longer as it lifts. To maintain the contact of the lifting leg with the shin bone of the "standing" foot, imagine that the moving leg is spreading mustard on a sandwich created by the shin bone of the standing foot and an imaginary wall just in front of the body. Additionally imagine a line of oppositional energy going out of the top of the head, and the ends of the toes pulling out into the space.

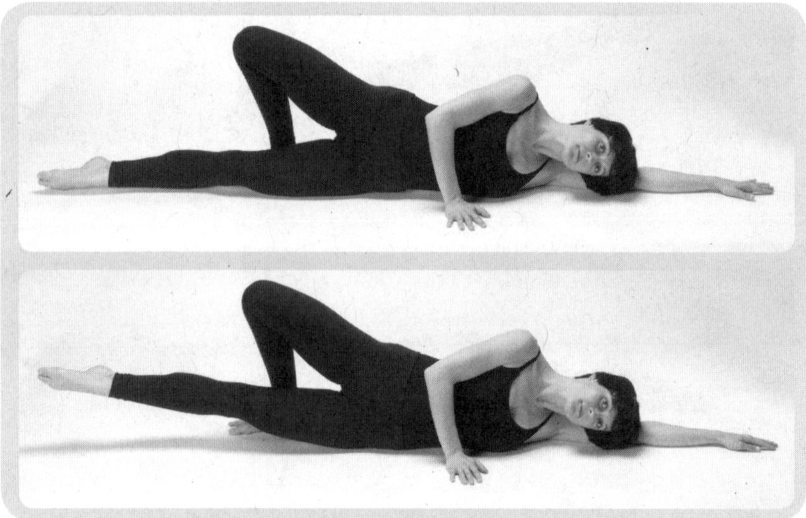

4) Dancing Legs (for Advanced Dancers)

(A) Développés on 3s: On count 1, reach the leg in a long arc until the inner legs touch with both feet pointed and reaching; on 2, bend the top knee and come to passé; on 3, extend the leg back to the side high position. Do four to eight repetitions.

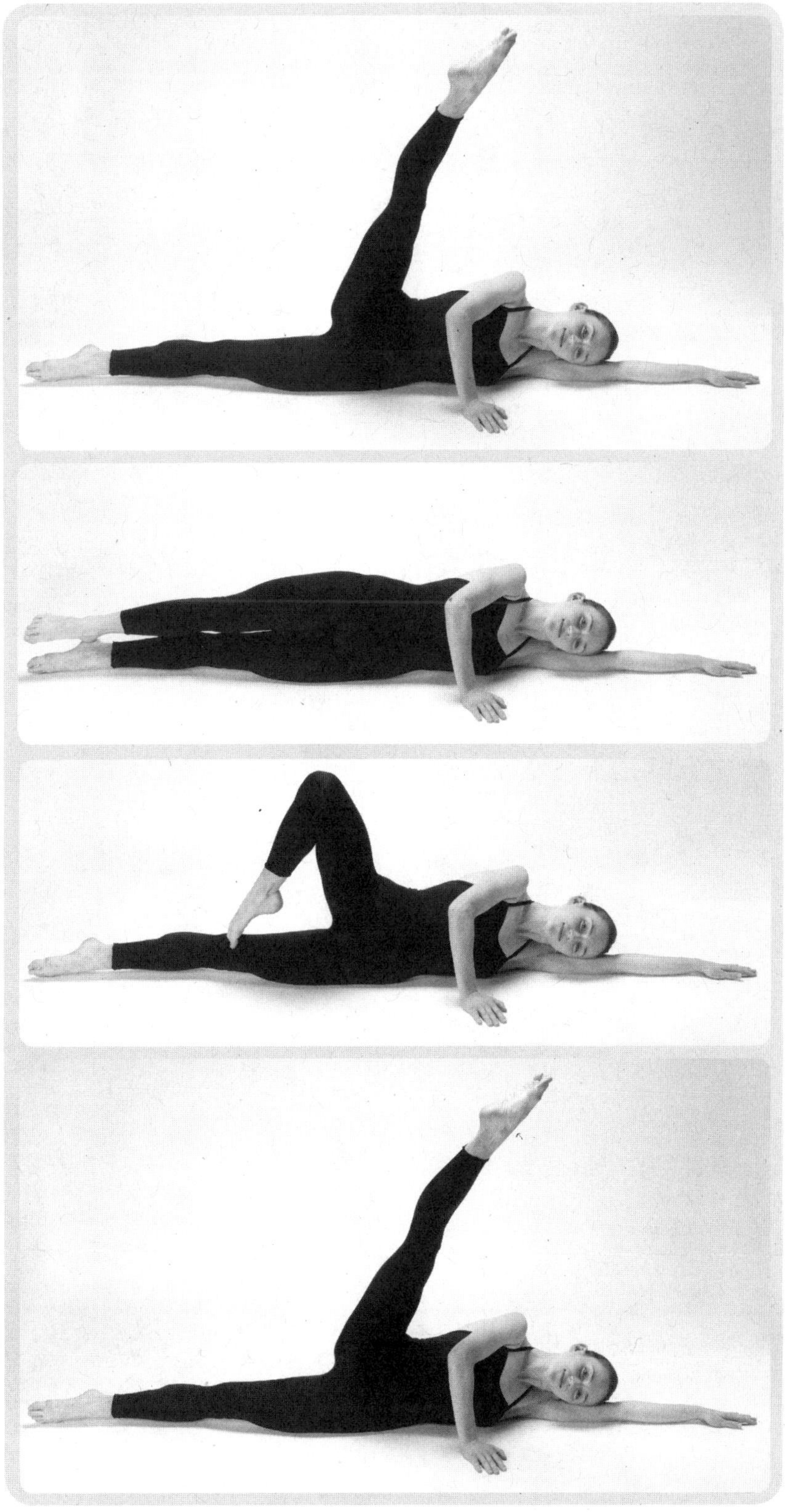

IMAGERY

For *Dancing Legs*, return to the image from the *Clam* of a stiff wire hanging from the ceiling that drops down through the top (right) hip socket and continues down through the bottom (left) hip into the floor. On count 1 of the développé and count 2 of the enveloppé, imagine the two legs joining together as if there is glue connecting the heels for an instant. On the high phase of each movement (count 3 of both directions), the leg should corkscrew up and out as it reaches, and energy should pour out of the foot. All of these images can also be used for the battements.

(B) Enveloppés on 3s: Reverse the direction, so that on count 1, bend the top knee and come to passé; on 2 extend the leg out along the bottom leg until the inner legs touch with both feet pointed and reaching; on 3, reach the leg directly up to the side high position, keeping the leg extended. Do four to eight repetitions.

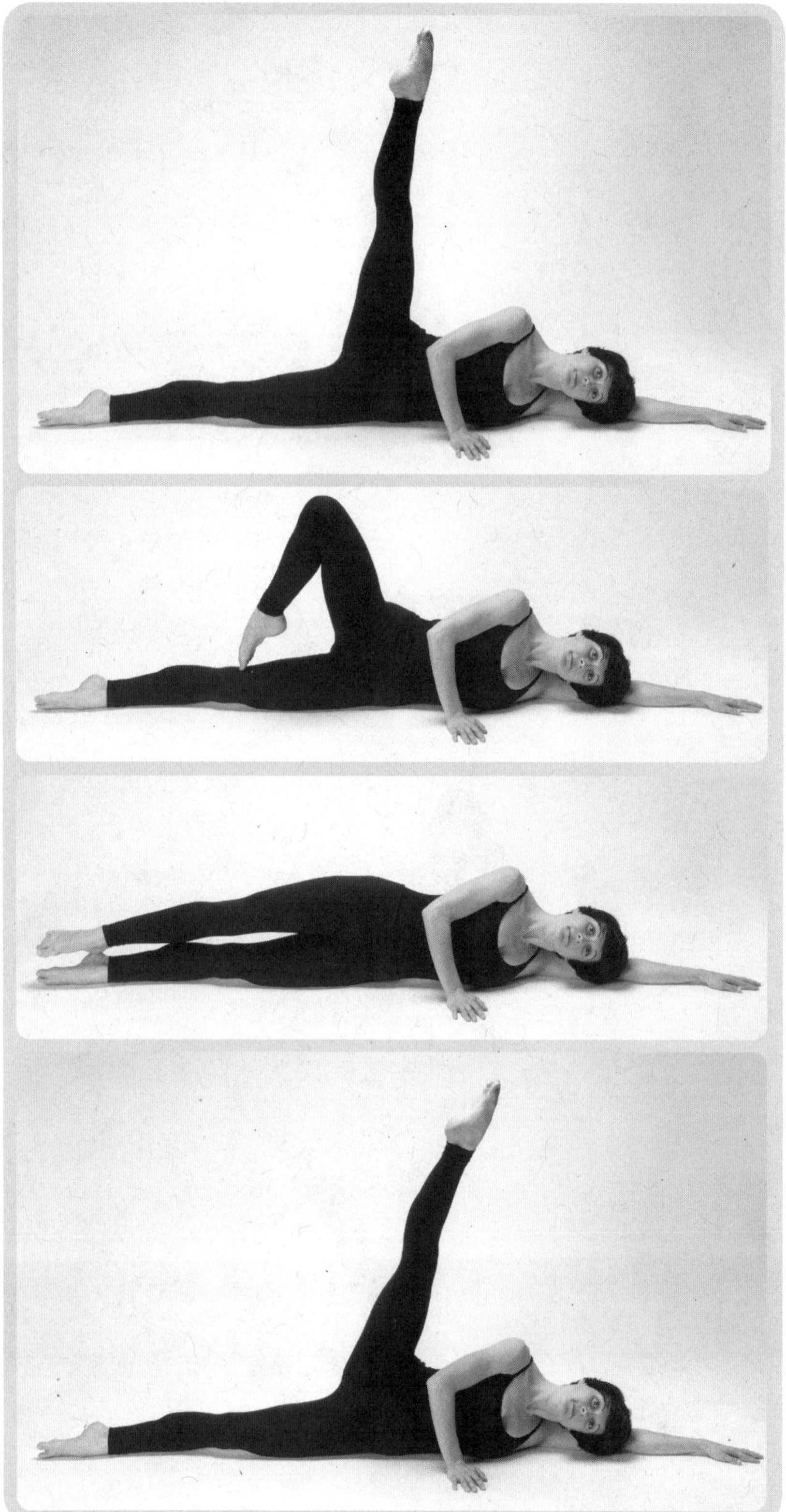

(C) Battements on 2s: On count 1, reach the leg in a long arc until the inner legs touch with both feet pointed and reaching; on 2, reach the leg directly up to the side high position, keeping the leg extended. Do four to eight repetitions.

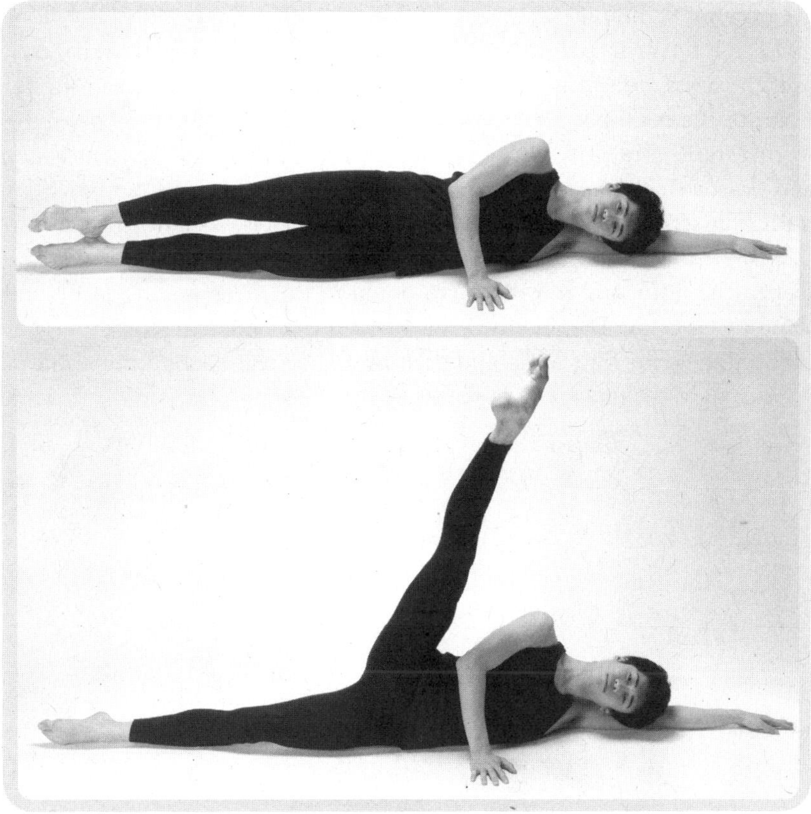

5) Spiral Stretch

Flex the foot, attempt to turn the hip out further, then lower the leg to the floor in front of the body for a spiral stretch. On the first side, take hold of the leg with the left hand moving the leg towards one o'clock on the clock, and reach the right arm (palm facing up) to a high diagonal at eleven o'clock, chest open to the ceiling. Focus to the right to complete the spiral. Relax for a thirty-second minimum stretch.

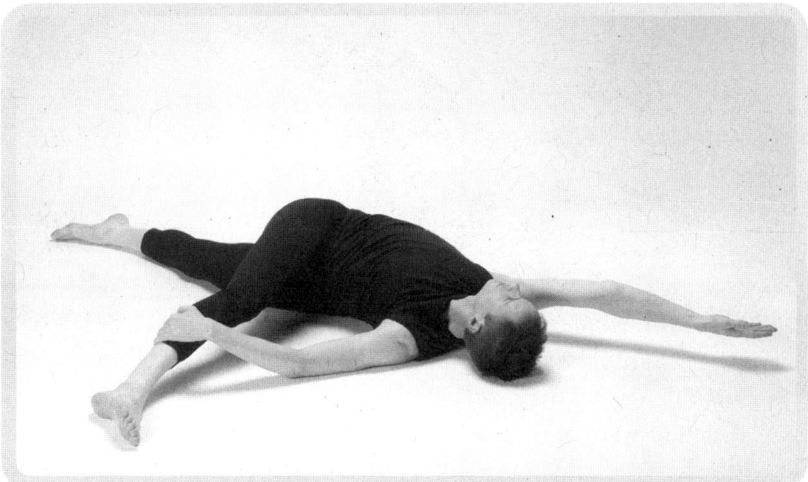

IMAGERY

For *Spiral Stretch*, allow the body to melt into the floor. See heat spreading from deep in the hips outward. With each exhale, allow the chest to widen and sink into the floor as the high diagonal arm becomes heavier.

6) Beats

In a fluid action, roll the sacrum to the floor and rond de jambe the right leg up to the ceiling, turning it out and pointing the foot. Développé the left leg to the ceiling, bringing the legs together. Flex the feet so they are now in "standing" first position. Lift the upper body off of the floor and reach the arms past the thighs, parallel to the floor in a rounded oval as if the arms are trying to encircle the legs. The top of the head should point to the ceiling with a space between the chin and chest. Lower the legs to the "point of control" (see Notes for Teachers on the next page), and do a series of beats in crossing fifth position at a brisk tempo. Start with four sets of eight beats, and build to eight sets of eight beats. Finish in first position; point the feet, rotate parallel, bend the knees, lower the feet to the floor, and roll the torso down to the floor, ending in neutral standing position. For an advanced variation, lift the legs slightly higher on the inhale for four beats, and then lower the legs back to the point of control on the exhale for four beats.

IMAGERY

For *Beats*, see the legs as tiny scissors slicing and cutting thin paper. Using the breath rhythm, deepen the hollowing on each exhale. As the legs are doing the *Beats*, the inner thighs are revolving towards the ceiling. Imagine trying to bring the hamstrings together. For the *Beats* with the hands clasped behind the head, imagine the inner surface of the elbow and upper arm reaching towards the thighs.

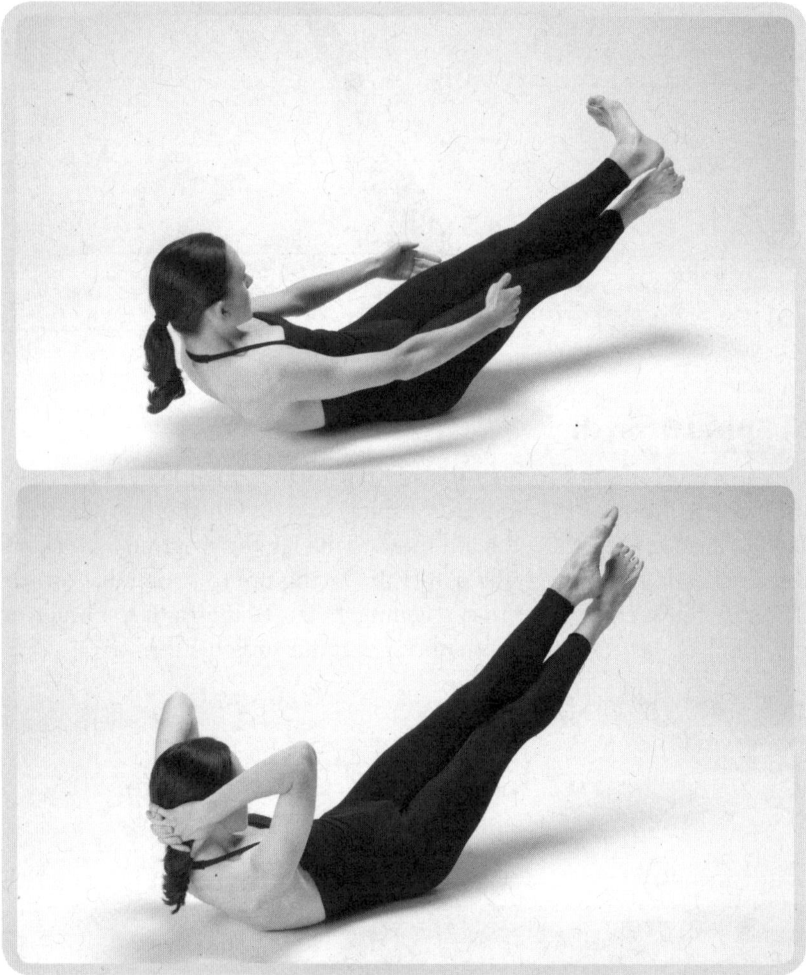

After the entire sequence is complete, repeat everything on the left side.

For the *Beats*, do the second side with pointed feet, and with the hands clasped at the back of the head.

At the conclusion of both sides, the dancers should extend the legs out along the floor and quietly rest.

Applications and Transfer to Standing and Travelling Work

As mentioned previously, this series challenges the core and the torso organization far more than the exercises performed while lying on the back, and prepares the dancer for the demands of working against gravity in stance. This series also assists the dancer in discovering the relationship of the femur to the torso for that particular individual's anatomical structure. This correct alignment of leg gesture to torso can assist in greater ease of movement as well as improved balance in adagio work. In the *Clam*, the problem of knee torque and implications for ligamentous laxity due to poor alignment were discussed. As the speed and range of motion increase (with movements such as développé and battements), the potential impact on the knees is greater. The negative consequences of wear and tear on the knee joints through repetitive twisting at the knee cannot be overemphasized.

Notes for Teachers

It is important to remind dancers to keep the top hip forward over the bottom hip throughout this entire series. Note: For most dancers, this means that the top leg will be in front of the pelvis and torso for all of the turned out work. Initially there will be considerable weight on the front hand, which will decrease as the dancers become stronger, particularly in the core support. If the dancers continue to struggle with this alignment, go back to working in pairs so the dancers can give each other support and feedback. Note: In both *Leg Lifts for the Outer Leg* and *Leg Lifts for the Inner Leg*, the work is in full range of motion, as long as the pelvis remains stable.

In *Leg Lifts for the Outer Leg*, the pelvis should remain entirely quiet, so that it is the femur moving in isolation, not the pelvis tilting, to lift the leg. The emphasis on the lift of the waist off of the floor will assist this action. At the end, on the last held lift, encourage the dancers to "turn in a little more!"

For *Pressing to the Back*, the image of the elastics is meant to encourage minimal release of the pelvis behind the body, so that the main action is hip extension (using the hamstrings and gluteus maximus), and not excessive arching of the lumbar spine. As in the exercise above, most of the movement should be the femur.

In *Leg Lifts for the Inner Leg*, dancers will most commonly want to place the femur in front of the pelvis, so that the hip flexors can contribute to the leg lift. It is important to remind them to maintain the lifting leg directly under the hip joint. If any of the dancers sickle the lifting foot, instruct them to lift the heel higher than the big toe as the leg is rising. Finally, if this position causes knee pain to the standing leg, or low back discomfort, place the standing leg in front of the lifting leg.

Dancing Legs is for advanced dancers only. It demands a high level of core support and organization to even attempt this series, so be willing to stay with the simpler side-lying work until the dancers are ready. When first introducing the développés, do eight repetitions of this first variation. As the other variations are added, limit the repetitions of each variation to four repetitions, because the total number of leg actions will continue to increase. The goal is to build strength without straining the muscles or causing excessive fatigue, especially if this work is done before or during class. As the dancers gain more control, the speed can be increased.

By the time the dancers get to the *Spiral Stretch*, it is not unusual for them to have a deep, burning sensation in the back of the hip. This is caused by the work of the deep external rotators, and can be quite intense at first. This stretch will release that tension, and give their hips a rest. The use of the high diagonal for the arm (rather than leaving the arm at shoulder height) releases the pectoralis minor muscle in the chest, which can cause round shoulders in dancers if it is tight.

In preparing for the *Beats*, the dancers begin by lowering the legs to the "point of control." This refers to the lowest point they can take the legs while still maintaining the low back in the slight undercurve (the *Bowl of the Body*, see page 27). The dancer should experience one long arc, like an empty bowl. If the dancer goes past the point of control, the low back will begin to arch. The beats should not be done with an arched spine, as it may cause injury to the low back.

The demand of these exercises can be increased by adding light weights to the ankles or by using elastic bands. These same exercises can be done standing with elastic bands, challenging balance while recruiting these important hip muscles.

PART SIX
ON EXTENSION

6

Opening Remarks

While some of the earlier work in C-I Training addresses muscles on the posterior aspect of the body (e.g., *Exercise on 6 for the Spine* on page 60, and *Pressing to the Back* on page 104), the focus of this section is to strengthen, recruit, mobilize, and integrate the muscles that contribute to the extension of the spine and legs. It is vital that the dancer understands the organization of the scapulae with the spine, and the integration of the legs with the core for work to the back (e.g., arabesque). Working prone in this series provides resistance for the work of the arms, and feedback for the pelvis in the connection to the floor. Additionally, research has suggested that strength work in extension of the spine can improve the height of the arabesque. Finally, the lumbar multifidi (deep lower back muscles) function with the transverse abdominal muscles in core support, and integrating these muscle groups—that is, learning to recruit them at the same time—can contribute to injury prevention work.

A – Supporting the Scapulae: Moving in the Sphinx

Purpose

The main purpose of this series is mobilization of the thoracic spine, and organization of the scapulae to support movements of the arms. While these ideas have been addressed previously, this series is far more challenging and demanding than previous work introduced in the *Arm Series on 8* (on page 19), or in *The Clock* (on page 31). *Massaging the Heart* specifically targets mobilizing the thoracic area for arches and arabesque work, as well as recruiting a muscle called the serratus anterior. This muscle connects the medial border of the scapula to the ribs and, if it is lacking in tone, can result in what is known as winged scapulae. In dancers that hold excess tension between the scapulae, the retreat phase can assist in releasing this tension. The purpose of *Shrugs – Descending Scapulae* is to strengthen and recruit the lower trapezius group for stabilization of the scapulae. Additionally, this exercise encourages core support in full arch of the lumbar spine. This is a progression from *Undercurves and Overcurves* (page 26) and from Variation 2 of the *Exercise on 6 for the Spine* (page 60). It is more challenging than these previous versions due to the length of time spent in the arch and this different relationship to gravity. The *Port de Bras* series connects the arms to the scapulae, and the scapulae to the spine and core, so that dancers are able to isolate movements of the arms during gestures without disrupting the quiet alignment of the scapulae and spine. Additionally, it requires supporting the weight of the torso on one arm, enhancing the strength of the arm for weight bearing.

IMAGERY

Throughout this series, whenever the spine is in the arched position off of the floor, imagine that the spine is like a Ferris wheel with energy coming out from the pelvis in a circular action, up and around. The back of the neck is very long and open, and the focus is straight out. Feel the circle of energy to keep the length in the back and reduce tension.

1) Sphinx

After completing A Trip Around the Hip, you will be lying on the back with the legs long. Roll over onto the front of the body and bring the upper torso up off of the floor, supporting the weight on the forearms. The elbows should be underneath the shoulders (not at the waist) and can be shoulder-width or slightly wider. Palms should be flat on the floor. Take some time to relax in this position, breathing fully into the ribs, and checking that the neck is long and easeful. Shoulders should be relaxed, as well as the legs and buttocks.

IMAGERY

For *Sphinx*, envision the Sphinx of Egypt, the grand recumbent lion waiting for eternity. One should embody both the weightedness and the serenity of this ancient mythical being.

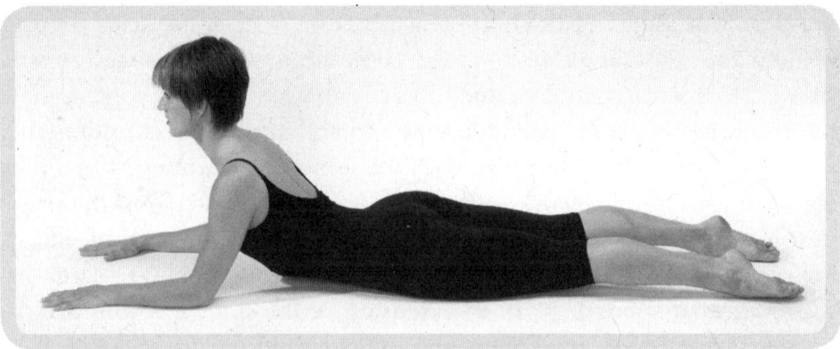

2) Massaging the Heart – Retreating and Advancing the Sternum

On four slow counts, push on the floor with the palms, and fully curl the thoracic spine, spreading the scapulae and retreating the sternum back between the scapulae. The head follows the line of the spine curve and drops down. Elbows and hips remain in contact with the floor. On counts 1,2, pull with the palms against the floor, and lengthen as much as possible through the lumbar spine; on 3, advance the sternum forward and extend the thoracic spine fully in an arc, projecting the sternum out into the space in front of the body; and on 4, lift the top of the head up as high as possible, eyes focusing straight ahead. Shoulders and neck remain easeful. Repeat four times.

IMAGERY

For *Massaging the Heart*, on the retreat, imagine the scapulae like broad wings opening and spreading across the back. On the advance, the pull of the hands should feel as if one is trying to drag oneself along the floor by the arms. Imagine the space between each of the lumbar vertebrae expanding to create the arch. As the sternum comes forward, sense a light from the heart bursting out of the sternum into the forward space. Imagine that the head is lifting high, as if growing Spock ears (*Star Trek*!).

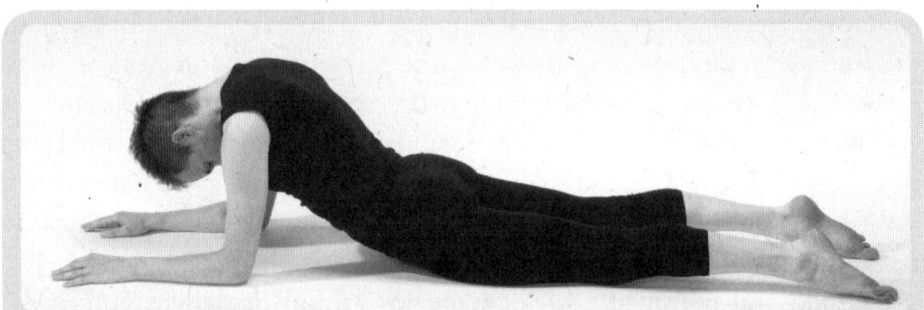

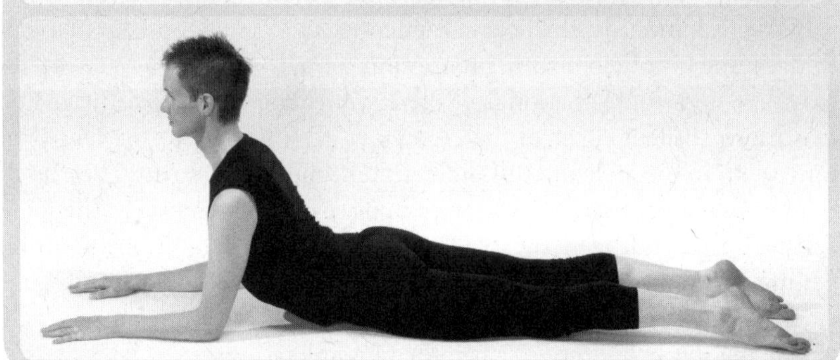

3) Shrugs – Descending Scapulae

Begin this series by elongating the elbows so that the weight is resting on the hands; do not bring the hands closer to the body. Allow the shoulders to come up around the ears (as in a shrug), letting the weight of the body drop towards the floor. The top of the head should remain towards the ceiling, although the neck will seem to disappear. Narrow and hollow, and then slowly slide the scapulae down the back towards the waist as the shoulders widen. Maintain and energize in this placement for about five seconds. Repeat this sequence three to four times.

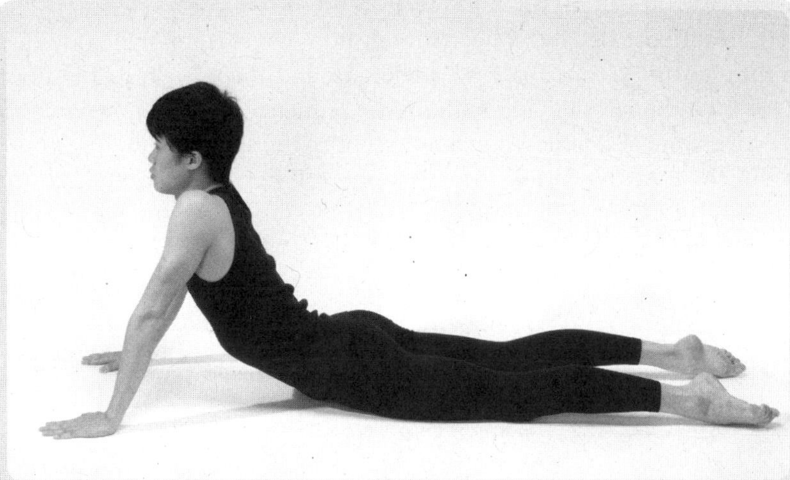

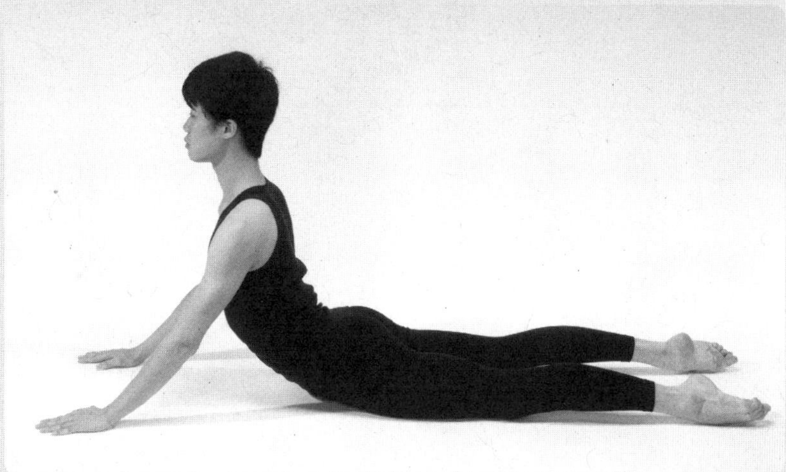

IMAGERY

For *Shrugs*, on the shrug, imagine the body as a scarecrow hanging on a pole. On the descent phase of the shoulders, imagine the scapulae as two slices of buttered toast. As the butter melts, the pieces of toast slide down the wall. Another image for *Shrugs* is that during the descent phase, the head is rising like a brave turtle out of its shell, then, as the shoulders return to the ears, the turtle retreats back into its shell.

4) Port de Bras

(A) Arabesque Arms: From the last *Shrugs – Descending Scapulae,* maintain the narrowing and hollowing, and reach the right arm into a long arabesque line in front of the shoulder, supporting the weight on the left hand. Try not to shift to the left. Place the right hand back down, and repeat on the left side.

(B) Arabesque Arm to High Fifth: Reach the right arm to arabesque line again, and then lift if up to fifth over the head, keeping the shoulder blade descending; reach the arm back to the arabesque line, and then place it back down on the floor. Repeat on the left side.

(C) Full Port de Bras: The arm will now travel from arabesque line, to fifth, out to second, back to arabesque, and then down to the floor. Repeat on the left side. Throughout the sequence, maintain or reinforce the narrowing and hollowing, the descent of the scapulae, and the width of the chest. At the end of the variations, roll slowly down through the spine and rest the forehead on stacked hands. Take some time to breathe, relaxing the back.

IMAGERY

For *Port de Bras*, imagine the energies of narrowing and hollowing, and of the sliding, descending scapulae as active ongoing movements to provide support for the arm gestures. Visualize the energy from the core and spine emanating out of the arms and hands in large circles. See the head continuing to float high.

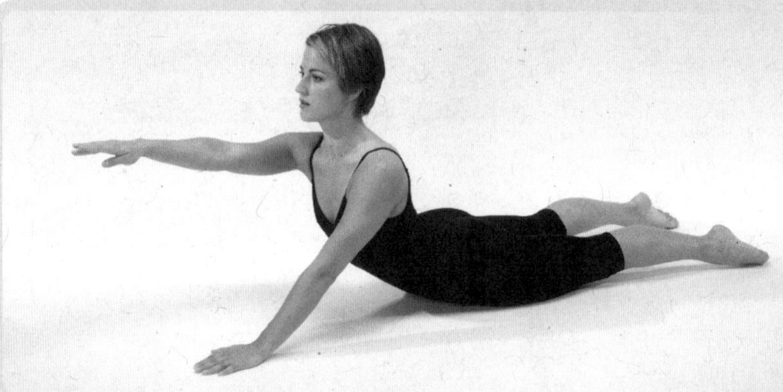

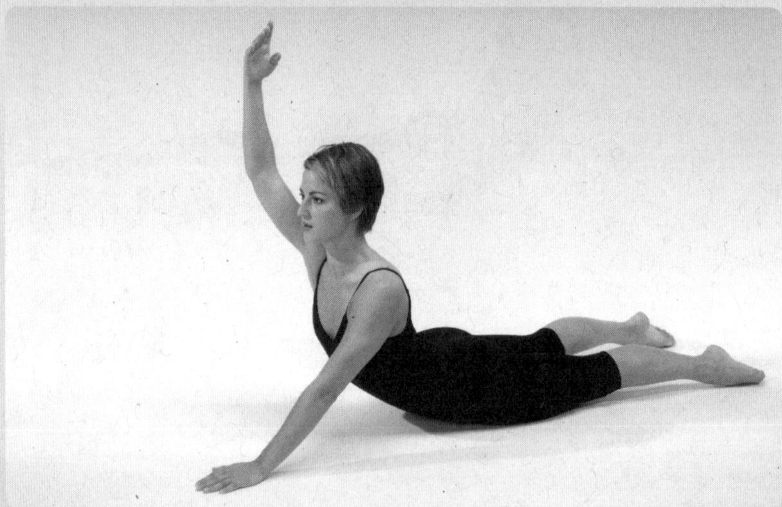

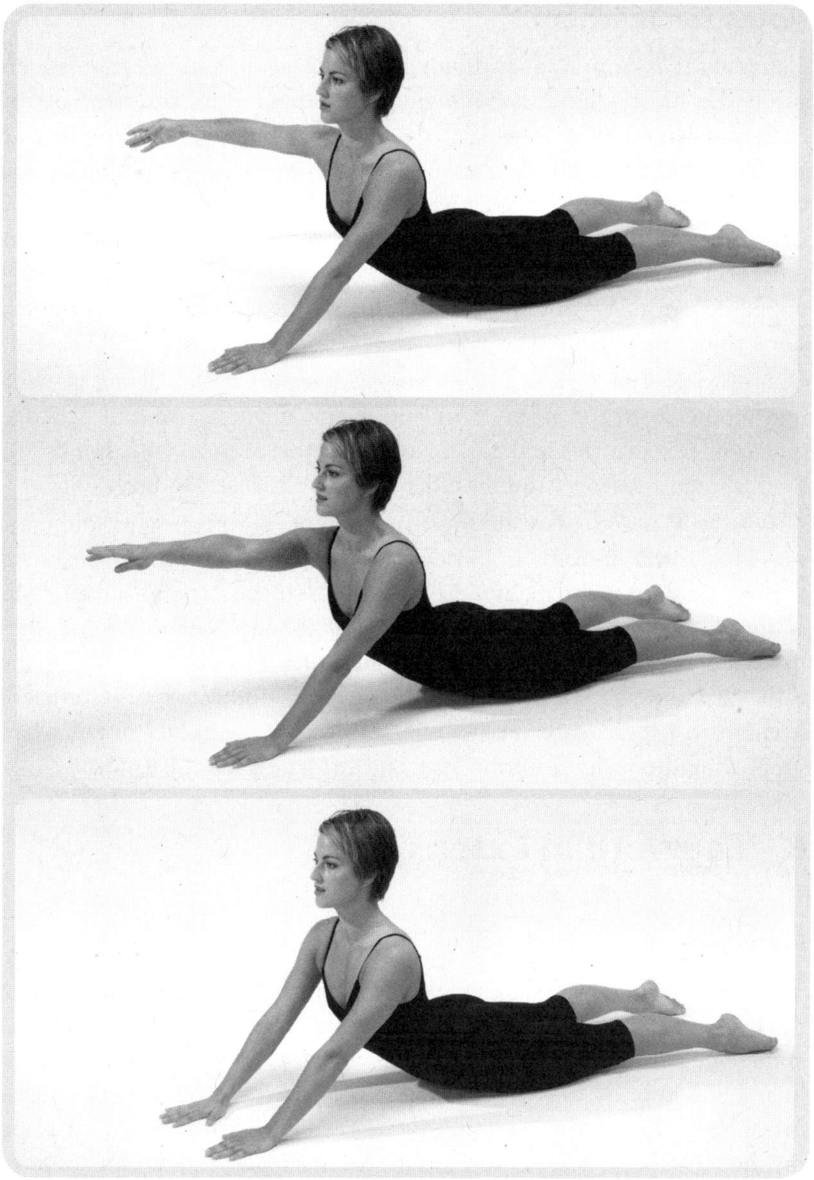

Applications and Transfer to Standing and Travelling Work

The paradox of the upper torso and arms in dance is that they require both tremendous mobility as well as unique stabilization. Although dance demands a large range of motion in arm gestures, it is one of the few forms that inhibits the forward movement of the scapulae (protraction) in forward-reaching gestures, and the elevation of the scapulae in high gestures. This need for arm mobility and scapular stability is addressed in this series. Further, arching the thoracic spine (an area of the spine with limited range in extension) is fundamental to many dance movements (arabesque, port de corps), and attention to this area is the centrepiece of this series. It should be noted that doing this arching work with the floor under the pelvis teaches to the dancer that when they stand and arch, the pelvis should not drift forward, but stay upright over the legs. Finally, the weight bearing on one arm can assist in preparing the arms for falls and partner work.

Notes for Teachers

Generally, it is important throughout this series to remind the dancers about the narrowing and hollowing, and about the alignment of the head and length of the neck. If dancers are struggling with retreating and advancing the sternum in *Massaging the Heart*, a gentle hand on the sternum can guide it backwards on the retreat, and encourage the sternum to reach forward on the advance. Note: In *Massaging the Heart*, the press phase involves simultaneous action of all the vertebrae and upper extremities, while the pull/reach phase is sequential, from lumbar spine to the head.

A possible stretch from the starting position for *Port de Bras* is to bend one elbow (e.g., the right arm) and rotate the torso to the opposite direction (e.g., to the left) for a passive stretch in arch with spiral. The focus should look over the shoulder towards the feet. Do both sides.

For the *Port de Bras*, relate these movements with actual standing and travelling dance movements, encouraging the dancers to use the focus as they would when dancing. Progress through the variations over time, as appropriate, or the back and shoulder joints can become strained. If the dancers are struggling with shoulder and scapular stability in the early variations, do not progress to the next one. Indicators of insufficient strength to progress are the inability to keep the shoulder down when supporting the weight on one arm, and struggling with balance.

B – Legwork in Extension

Purpose

This series consists of strength work for all of the posterior muscles of the legs and upper limbs, as well as the lumbar spine. Additionally, it can encourage core support for legwork to the back, and for torso movement in arches and body rolls, if the awareness of narrowing and hollowing is maintained during the sequences. The series is also designed to teach turnout in extension, and to educate the motor system about some of the accommodations that need to be made to achieve a full arabesque. The feedback from the floor can encourage the correct motor control in the standing leg, working the extensors of that leg (the hamstrings) as well as turnout and inner thigh activity. Finally, the series encourages the alignment of the scapulae and upper limbs in this full body organization for arabesque work.

Inadequate core support and poor alignment in leg and torso work in extension can result in injuries to the lumbar spine, particularly in the adolescent dancer. This series can offer strategies for injury prevention through both muscular strength and neuromuscular patterning. The emphasis on inner thigh work can assist in developing muscle balance between the outer and inner thighs, contributing to a healthier mechanism in knee action.

1) Double Leg Extensions

Lying prone, with the hands under the forehead, bring the legs to parallel with the feet slightly apart, directly in line with the sitz bones. Fully dorsiflex the ankles and curl the toes under so that they are in contact with the floor. The knees are bent and completely relaxed. On counts 1,2,3, extend the legs by reaching out in the space with the heels and keeping the front of both hips in contact with the floor; on 2,2,3, relax the knees back down to the floor again. Repeat eight times, remaining in the last extension. Point the feet, keeping the thighs off of the floor and the legs extended. Slowly lower the legs back to the floor, maintaining the parallel alignment of the hip joints.

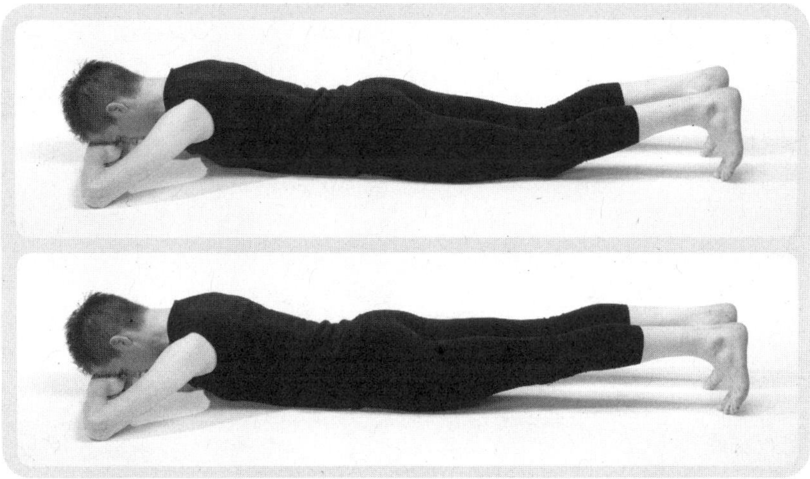

IMAGERY

In *Double Leg Extensions*, imagine that it is the reach of the heels into the space that causes the legs to elongate, rather than the action of straightening the knees. Visualize a wall that the heels are pushing against as they move away from the pelvis. Imagine that the ASIS bones in the front of the pelvis are glued to the floor and cannot lift off the ground, and the plane formed by the ASIS bones and pubic bone lies parallel to the floor. See a line of energy from the sitz bones to the heels, and sense a connection along this line of energy, even though the heels are moving away from the pelvis.

2) Parallel Alternating Leg Lifts

Lift one leg at a time, initiating the lift by first elongating the leg along the floor on "and," and then lift it off the floor, reaching out in the space 1; lower the leg back down to the floor 2. As in the *Double Leg Extensions*, the front of both hips remain on the floor. Alternate legs, so that there is a total of eight lifts. Transition: Lift both legs off the floor 1; turn them out, bring the heels together on 2; lower the legs to the floor on 3; and bring the arms to a high V on the floor, reaching out from the shoulder joints on 4.

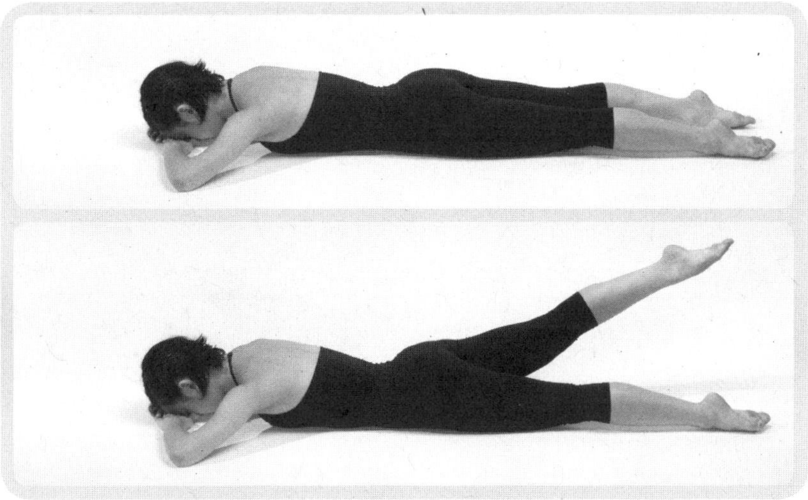

IMAGERY

In *Parallel Alternating Leg Lifts* and *Turned Out Alternating Leg Lifts*, imagine that the leg gets longer and longer with each lift. Imagine that there is an increase in the space inside the hip socket, so that the leg is literally moving away from the pelvis. The front of the hip is taffy, and it stretches out to allow the lift of the leg. The shoulder blades continually melt down towards the waist, which is narrowing and hollowing throughout the series. Even as the arm lift is added, the shoulder blades are connected to the waist, and the space from the shoulder to the ear elongates.

3) Turned Out Alternating Leg Lifts

Repeat the same leg action as described in *Parallel Alternating Leg Lifts*, elongating the leg along the floor and, lifting it off the floor on 1, while at the same time lifting the opposite arm so that as the right leg lifts, the left arm lifts off the floor; lower the leg back down to the floor on 2, making sure the heels and inner thighs touch, and lower the arm to the floor back to the high V. Note: The leg is directly in line with the hip joint, and the arm is on a diagonal in the line of pull of the latissimus dorsi muscle; that is, at one o'clock and eleven o'clock if the body is lying in the centre of a clock. The forehead and hips remain on the floor, so that the limbs are isolated in the action. Alternate legs so that there is a total of eight lifts.

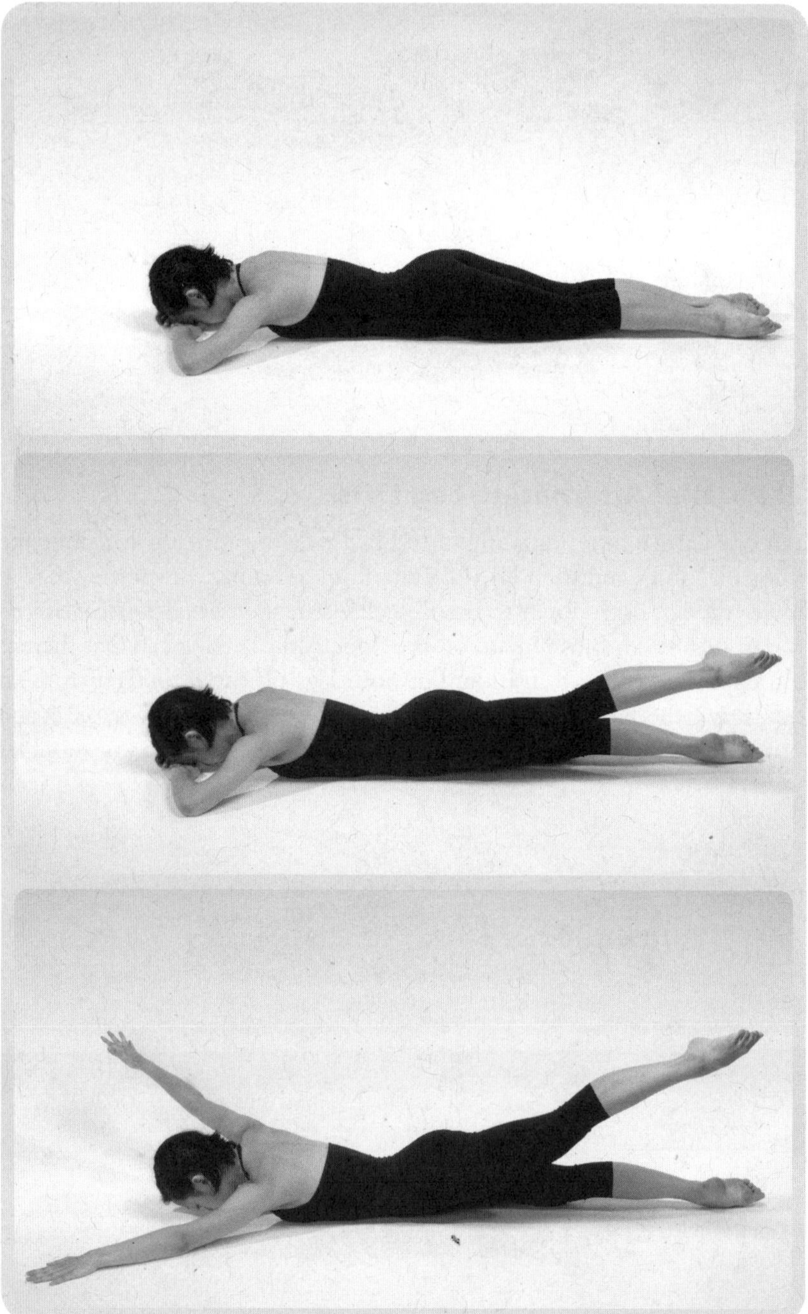

Variation 1 – Flexing the Foot: On count 1, lift the leg and opposite arm. On 2, flex the foot and reach out the heel. On 3, point the foot. And on 4, lower the leg back down to the floor.

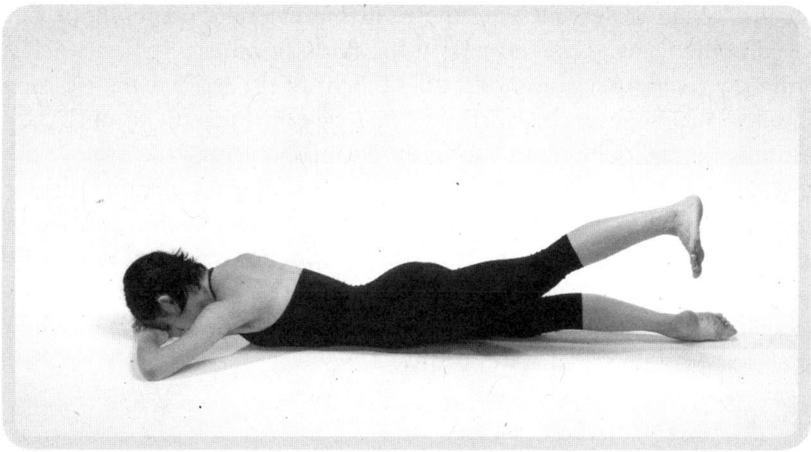

Variation 2 – Bending the Knee: On count 1, lift the leg and opposite arm; on 2, bend (flex) the knee, bringing the leg to a low back attitude; on 3, extend the knee and reach the leg out in the space again; on 4, lower the leg back down to the floor. Note: Variations A and B can be done without the arm lift, to allow the dancer to focus on the leg action and pelvic stabilization.

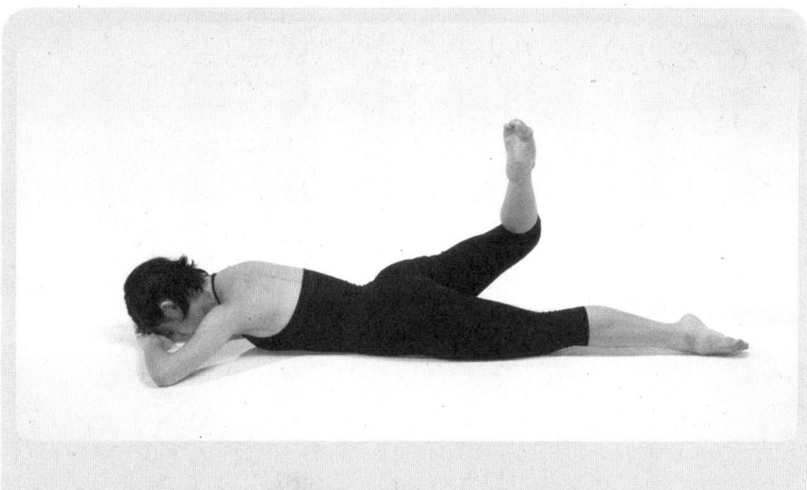

4) Exercise on 6 for the Arabesque

Bring the hands back under the forehead. On count 1, slide the right leg along the floor and lift it as in *Turned out Alternating Leg Lifts* above. On 2, lift the leg higher by allowing the right hip to come off the floor, but keeping the front of the left hip on the floor. In other words, the pelvis will now rotate to accommodate the height of the leg, but the rib cage should remain entirely on the floor. On 3, flex the knee to 90° or slightly more, wrapping the leg to a back attitude and elongating the front of the thigh. On 4, extend the leg back to the arabesque again (taking it higher if possible) without displacing the left hip. The right foot should be in alignment directly behind the right shoulder, and not opened out to the side or over-crossed. On 5, lower the right hip back to the floor, trying to keep as much height in the leg as possible. On 6, lower the leg back to the floor, bringing the heels together.

IMAGERY

Visualize the standing arabesque while doing *Exercise on 6 for the Arabesque*. The pelvis is rotating, but the standing hip remains turned out and open (long) in the front. The rib cage rotates in the opposite direction to stay "square" in relation to its spatial orientation. The upper body stays relaxed but energized, with the lumbar spine elongating as the leg reaches out in the space. The inner thighs and heels connect each time the leg closes back to first position.

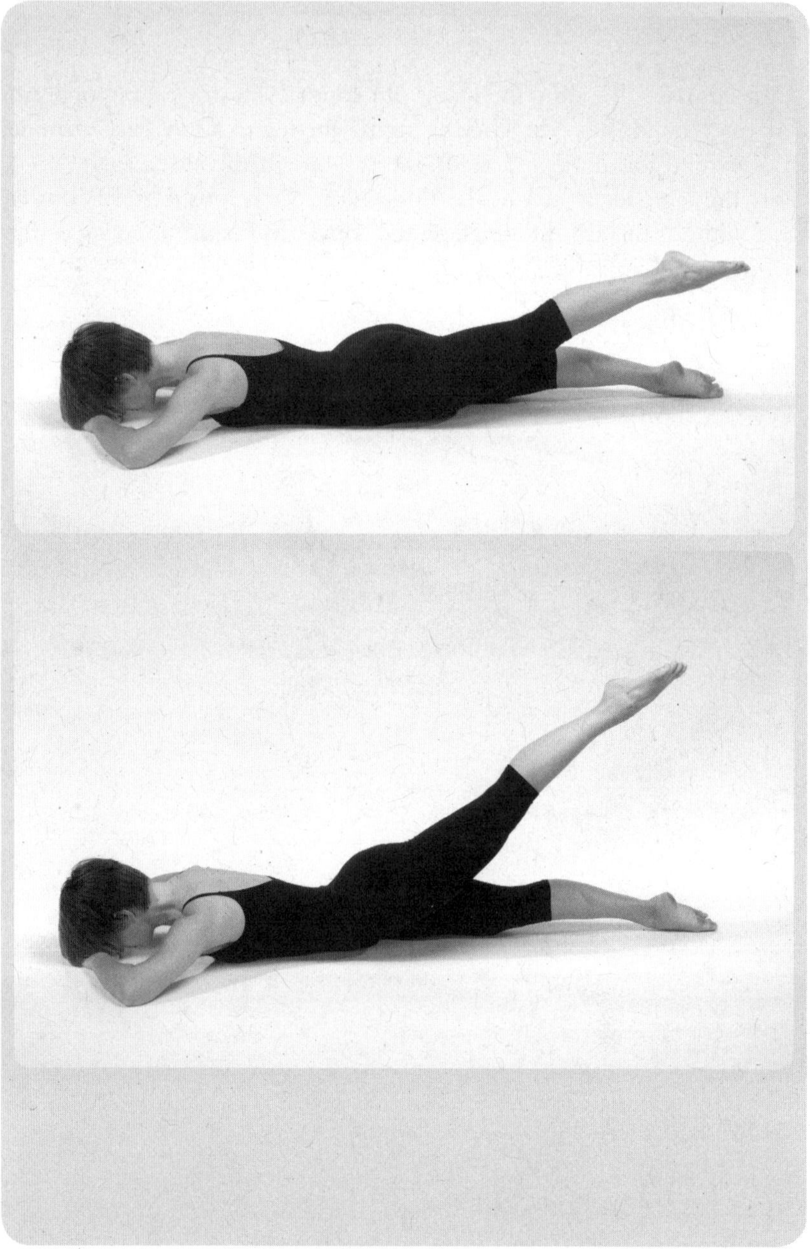

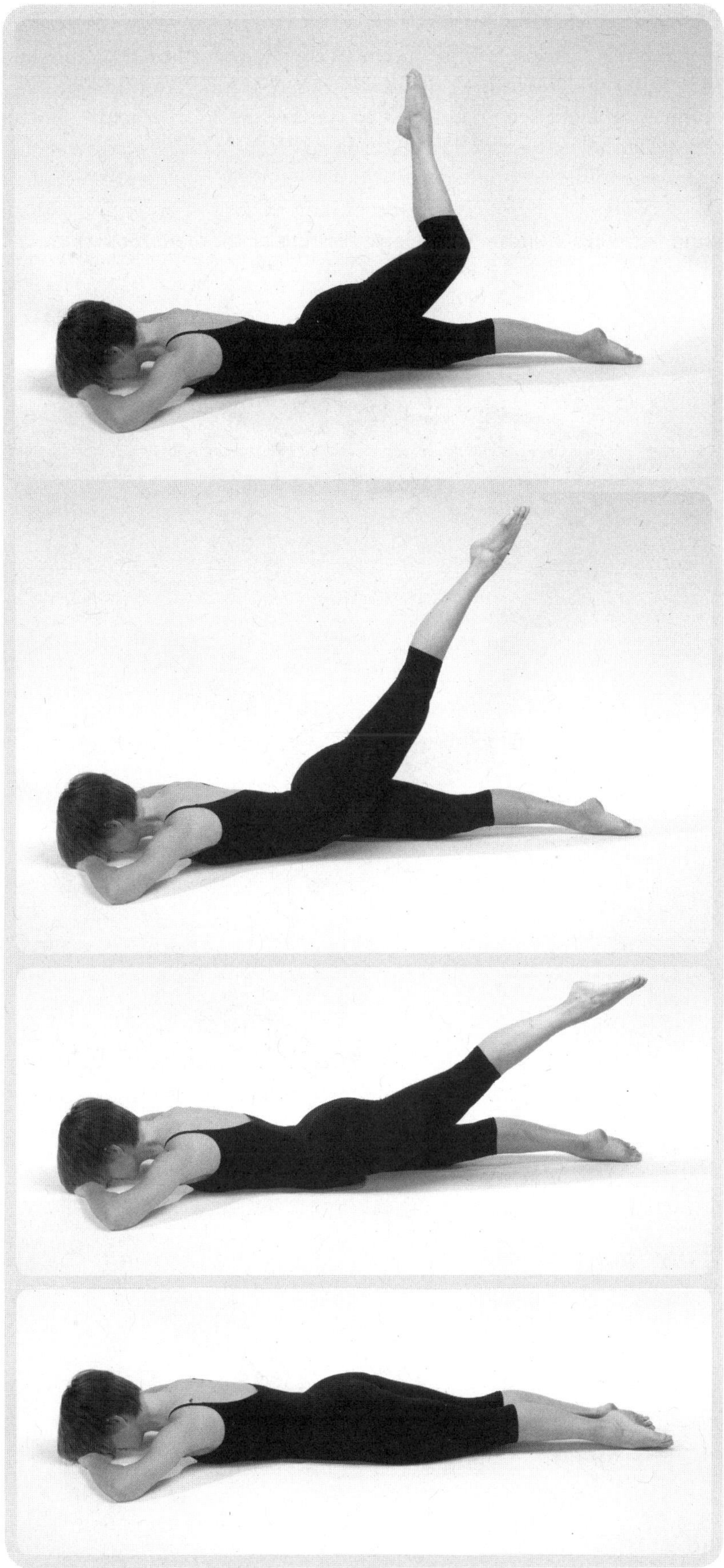

5) Beats in Low Arabesque

Bring both legs just off the floor, heels together, hips remaining on the floor. On a very fast 4, do small beats of the heels in first position, completing eight sets of 8-4s. Keep the legs and feet reaching out in the space throughout. Repeat with flexed feet. As the dancers become stronger, another set pointed and another set flexed can be completed. At the end, do a small hollowing or scooping of the low back (like a small contraction) to elongate and release the muscles of the lumbar spine.

IMAGERY

In *Beats in Low Arabesque*, imagine the legs like tiny scissors cutting paper behind the body. Another useful image is that of red slippers on the feet as in *The Wizard of Oz*, clicking the heels together to go back home.

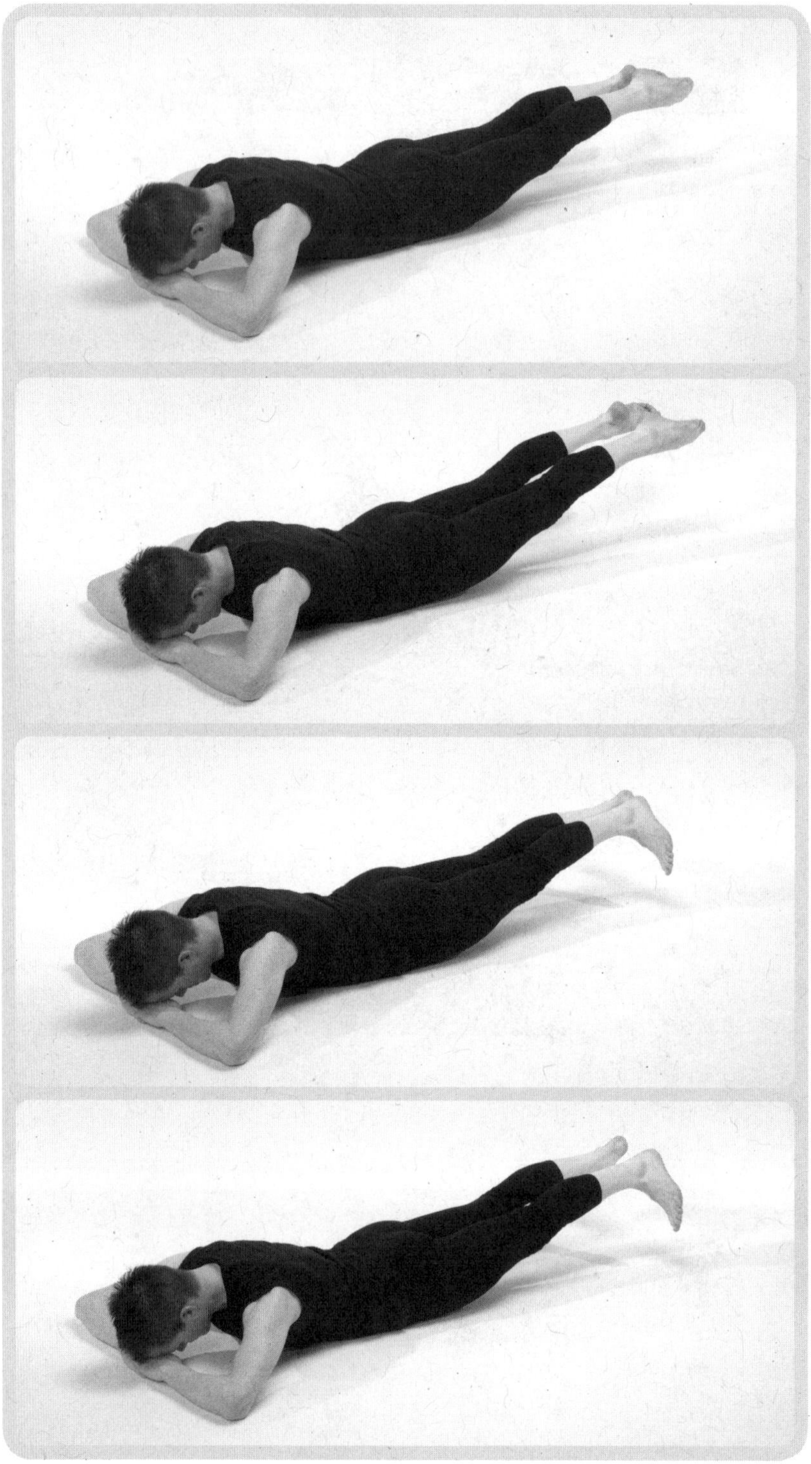

Applications and Transfer to Standing and Travelling Work

As stated above, this series relates directly to standing and travelling legwork in extension, from tendu to arabesque and grand battement. The coordination and organization of the trunk for these movements is complex. The sensation of sliding the leg along the floor before it lifts in both parallel and turned out leg lifts relates directly to the sensation of reaching the foot down and out to initiate a tendu, not starting the tendu by tilting the pelvis. Note: The one major adjustment that cannot occur while lying prone is the motion of the upper torso moving forward, which is necessary when standing, as the leg goes to full height towards the back. This will limit the leg height in this series, and the importance of this adjustment in stance should be pointed out to the dancers.

Notes for Teachers

It is very useful to teach the *Double Leg Extensions* in pairs. Firstly, the partner can actually hold the heels and gently pull the heels out, guiding them in space away from the pelvis. Secondly, the partner can gently place the palms of the hands on the heels to suggest the pressing of the heels into the space. Remind the dancers to keep the hips firmly attached to the floor or the pelvis will tend to go into anterior tilt and create a lumbar arch (swayback).

As the legs begin to come off of the floor in the remaining exercises in this series, continue to reinforce the idea of space in the hip joints and length of the legs. Some dancers may be too tight in the hip flexors to achieve any lift of the leg without the hips coming off of the floor. Dancers with this inflexibility should be strongly encouraged to do daily hip flexor stretching, as it indicates that they will be creating their arabesque line entirely from spine extension—a potential cause of low back problems.

Note: The *Exercise on 6 for the Arabesque* is very advanced. Dancers will be able to accomplish the other exercises in this series long before they should attempt *Exercise on 6 for the Arabesque*. If the dancers cannot maintain the connection of the standing hip to the floor and/or if they cannot sustain a clear spatial orientation with the arabesque leg even with coaching and imagery, then it may be too soon for them to attempt this exercise.

Finally, many dancers will begin to exhibit tension in the neck and shoulders from the intensity of this series. Keep encouraging relaxation of the upper body through awareness and imagery.

C – The Ferris Wheel: The Spine in Extension

Purpose

The purpose of this series is to strengthen the extensors of the spine. With so much emphasis today on abdominal work, it is easy to forget that the posterior muscles are also important, and the deep spine extensors contribute to core support and injury prevention. Additionally, this series addresses the scapular adductors and depressors (rhomboids and lower trapezius muscles), which are crucial to the stabilization of the scapulae for the dancer's line, that is, maintaining the shoulders wide and dropped to accentuate the line of the neck and chest. Finally, at the end of the Chest Lift series (#1-4), the egg breathing exercise allows the dancer to experience posterior/lateral breathing, which is often blocked by the bracing and tension dancers carry in the back.

1) Chest Lifts on 3s Plain

Still lying prone, bring the arms to the sides of the body with the hands next to the hips, palms facing down and touching the floor; the forehead is on the floor. On counts 1,2,3, lift the upper body into an arch, initiating the movement by reaching the top of the head out along the floor and then up off the floor on 1, followed by the shoulder area on 2, and, finally, the chest on 3. The action is circular and continuous, with the back of the neck and upper spine elongating. On 2,2,3, reverse the action, lowering the chest, then the shoulders, and then the head, forehead returning to the floor so the back of the neck remains long. Repeat four times.

IMAGERY

For this entire series, the image of the spine as a Ferris wheel is excellent, as it assists in keeping the spatial intention of the motion circular and elongated. Visualize the top of the head reaching out and up.

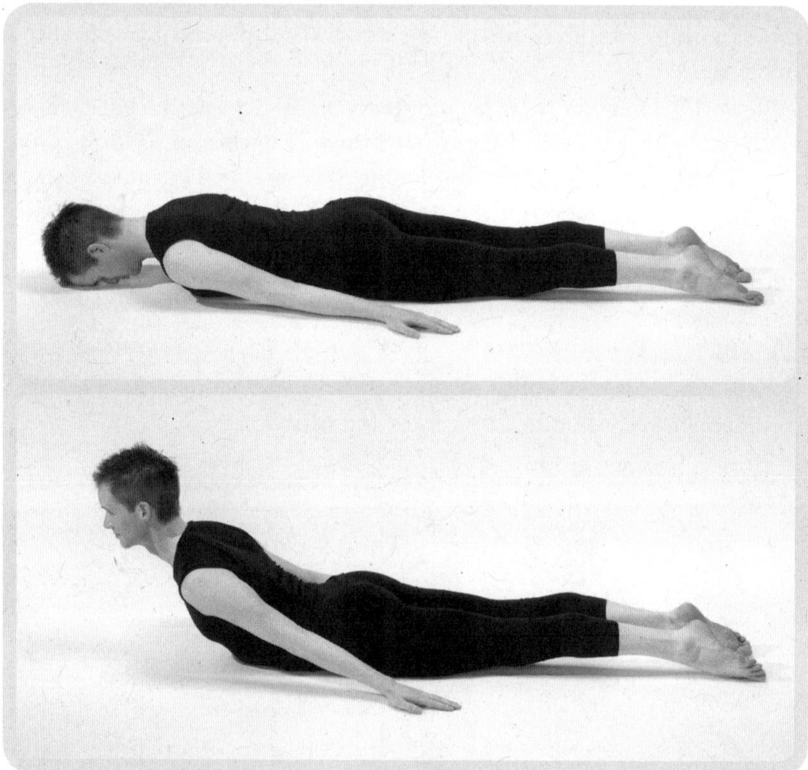

2) Flying Bird – Chest Lifts on 3s with Arms Behind

For *Flying Bird*, the action of the spine is the same as in the previous exercise, but now the arms come off the floor as high as the shoulders and reach behind the body. The shoulder blades come together for this variation, but do not lift up towards the ears or back of the head. Palms remain facing down, and the arms are long but easeful. Arms return to the floor each time the body lowers. Repeat four times.

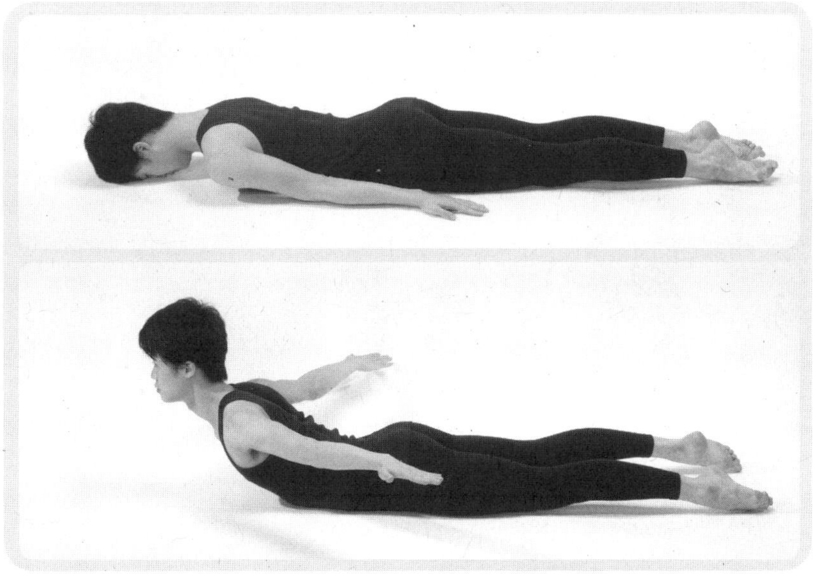

IMAGERY

For *Flying Bird*, imagine the scapulae being drawn together like two magnets, the arms like the wings of a bird helping to lift the body away from the floor. See the chest widen and reach forward as if leaning into the wind.

3) Widening the Back – Chest Lifts on 3s with Arms in Second

Bring the arms directly out to the side of the shoulders, resting on the floor, palms down. The action of the spine is repeated, this time with the arms lifting to classical second position. Both the chest and the back remain wide in this variation, and the arms should be visible to the dancer. Arms return to the floor each time the body lowers. Repeat four times.

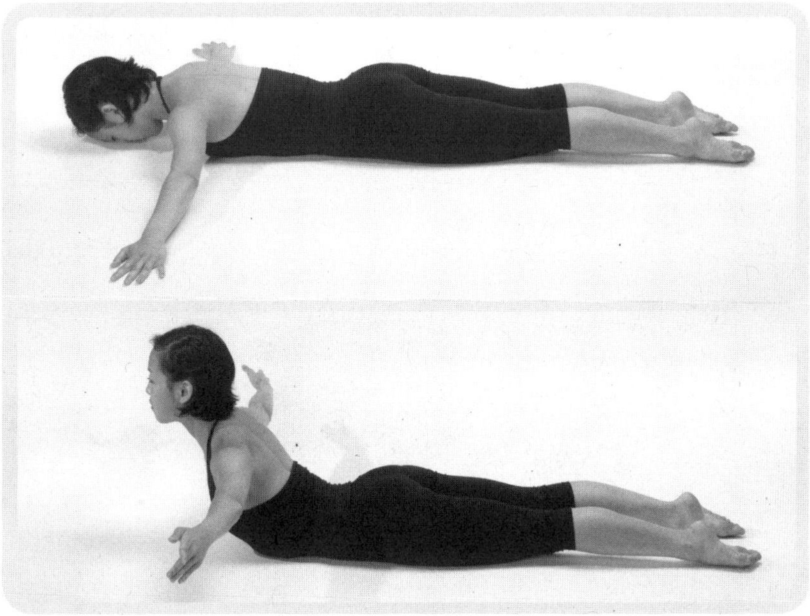

IMAGERY

For *Chest Lifts on 3s with Arms in Second* and *Chest Lifts on 3s with Arms in Fifth*, imagine the back lengthening and widening at the same time, and the arms as gorgeous circles embracing space. See the scapulae sliding down towards the waist, like the toast with melting butter from *Shrugs* (on page 113).

4) Final Strength Work – Chest Lifts on 3s with Arms in Fifth

Bring the arms to fifth position, resting on the floor. The action of the spine is repeated once more, this time with the arms lifting to fifth overhead. Shoulders should remain dropped, with the scapulae melting down towards the waist, the neck long and elegant. Arms return to the floor each time the body lowers. Repeat four times. At the end, hold the last lift, bring the feet just off the floor, turn out the legs, point the feet, and reach the energy out in all directions.

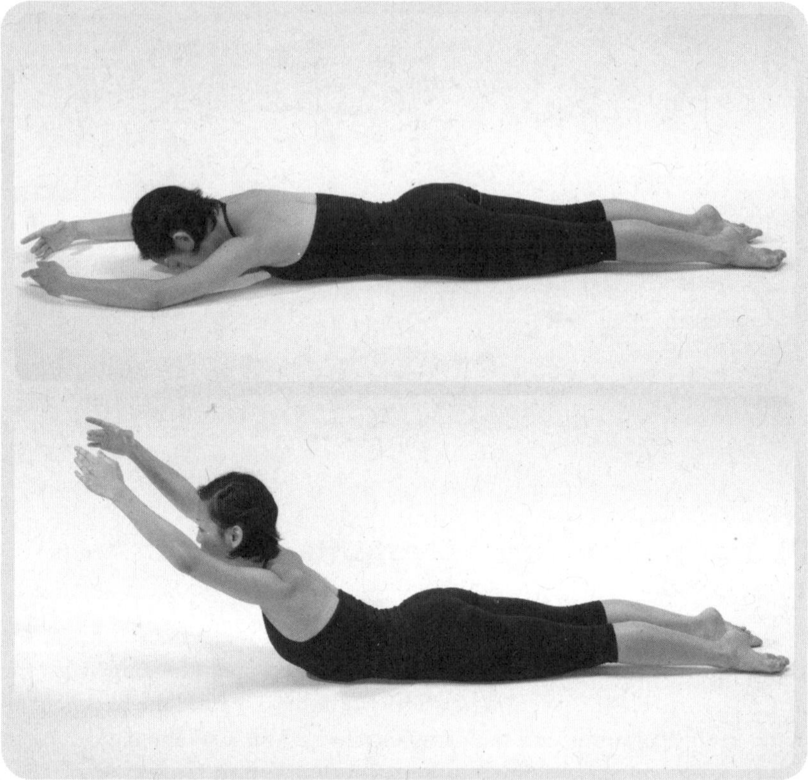

5) Final Rest – Egg Stretch

Pull back into an egg shape, sitz bones resting on the heels, forehead to the floor, and arms at the sides of the body with the hands near the feet. Allow the scapulae to drop apart, and breathe into the sides and back of the rib cage.

IMAGERY

For *Egg Stretch*, see the whole body breathing and expanding, with air filling the ribs, pelvis, and lumbar area. Imagine the scapulae heavy, weighted, and sliding around the rib cage towards the floor.

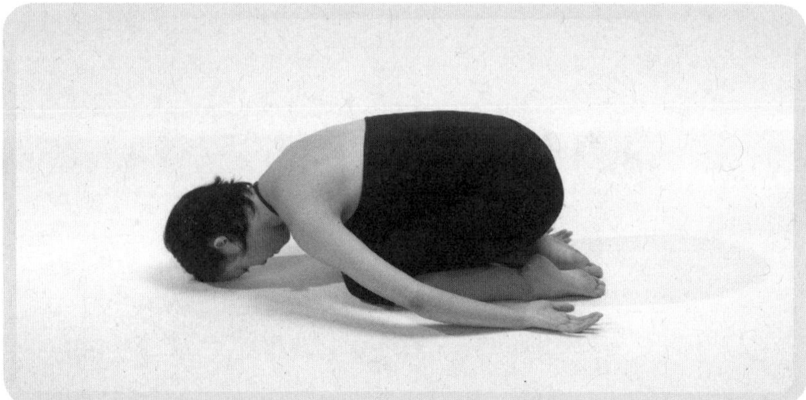

Applications and Transfer to Standing and Travelling Work

This series can assist in all standing and travelling material that demands strength in the extensors of the spine. Extensor strength can aid in improved height of arabesque, as well as reduced risk of injury in partnering work and weight-sharing material in choreography. Additionally, the attention to the rhomboids and lower trapezius muscles assists in dance-related aesthetics for use of the arms with scapular stabilization. Thinking of the line of the spine in arches and arabesque as a Ferris wheel can encourage the length of the spine and space between the vertebrae. It can also help distribute the arching motion throughout the spine rather than keeping it entirely in the lumbar area.

Notes for Teachers

Remind the dancers that the legs should remain as relaxed as possible. It is not important in this series that the legs be completely together, or that they be fully extended. The focus is for the upper torso. Some of the very flexible dancers will want to arch all the way into the lumbar spine in these chest lifts, but the focus is more for the thoracic area. The lumbar area should remain on the floor. Even lifting just to the twelfth thoracic vertebra will activate the lower deep extensors; it is not necessary to arch higher than T12. Build this series progressively; make sure that the dancers are achieving *Chest Lifts on 3s Plain* easily before moving on to the remaining variations. It may take several weeks before the dancers can do all of the variations. If the dancers are having problems breathing in the *Egg Stretch*, have them work in pairs. One partner can place the palms of the hands gently on the posterior/lateral rib cage of the partner in the egg, and the person in the egg can imagine trying to fill the hands with air from the lungs.

7 PART SEVEN FINAL STRENGTH AND STRETCH

Opening Remarks

This last section of C-I Training incorporates a final strength exercise with core support (a series of stretches repeated from Part Three – Flexibility Series) and work to develop proprioception and balancing mechanisms. The final stretches and balancing work also serve as a transition to stance, allowing some time for the dancer to organize the body in neutral, energized alignment in upright posture.

Purpose

This final sequence provides a strength exercise for the upper limbs, which demands core support, and final stretches to address flexibility in areas of the body—hip flexors, calves, hamstrings, and spine—that are essential for dancers. Even when working correctly, dancers can find that these areas become tight and tense from the overuse of these muscles in dance practice. Tightness in these areas can lead to poor alignment, tension patterns, and injuries.

Rolling Up to Stance and *Balancing Work* with eyes closed serve as awareness exercises and proprioceptive training. Dancers can become almost exclusively visually dependent, especially with the emphasis on use of mirrors in dance training, and due to the focus on upright work in many dance forms. Taking away vision for balances compels the motor system to rely on proprioceptive input for balance, and can assist in improving this mechanism for balance control. Further, taking the time to focus mentally on dynamic alignment (that is, with the body moving rather than stationary) can provide useful information and tools for sensing and enhancing one's alignment in dance.

1) Push-Ups

Begin by coming to all fours (hands and knees). Take some time to find the length of the neutral spine and to narrow and hollow. The head should be in line with the spine, with the focus on the floor in front of the hands. If the focus is between the hands or under the torso, the head will tend to hang down. Hands should be shoulder width or slightly wider. Flex the right foot and extend the right leg directly out behind the body, placing the foot on the floor. Then do the same action with the left foot, so that the body is now in one long line from head to heels, in a push-up position. In a controlled action, on count 1, lower the chest to the floor, keeping the pelvis in line; that is, not flexing at the hip joints or dropping the pelvis to the floor. On 2, press back up into the beginning position without locking or popping into the elbow joints.

Repeat four to sixteen times. Variation – Scapular Push-Ups with Plank: Come to the push-up position as described above. Keeping the elbows extended, lower the body towards the floor by allowing the scapulae to draw together. Then push away from the floor by moving the scapulae apart (abduction or protraction) as far as possible. This is the same action that the scapulae do in *Massaging the Heart* (see page 112). The trunk remains extended, head in alignment. Do four repetitions in eight slow counts. Stay in the extended (plank) position for eight more counts. Do two complete sets. For added difficulty, do a third and fourth set balanced on one foot, with the other foot at the back of the supporting ankle.

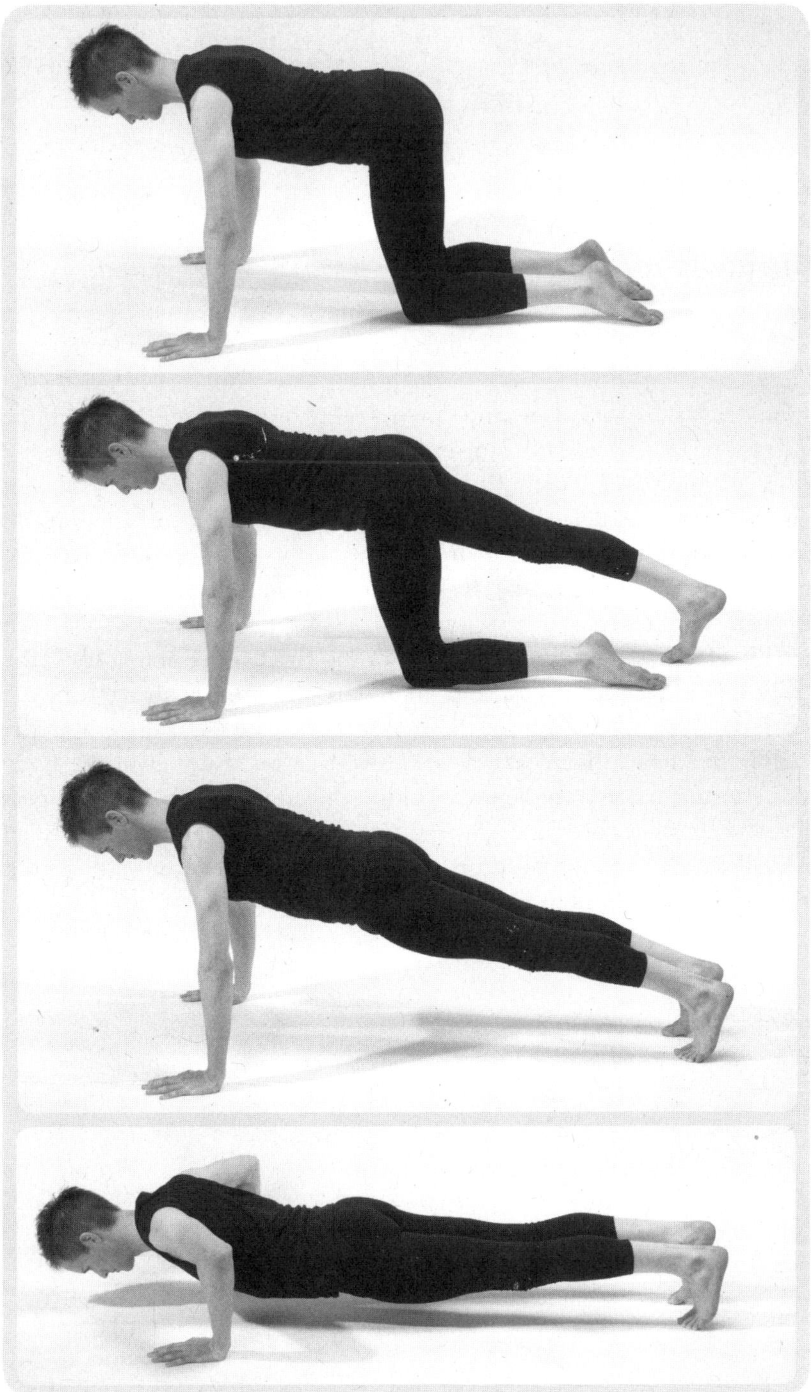

IMAGERY

For *Push-Ups*, imagine a line of energy going out of the top of the head and the heels in opposite directions. Only the elbows and shoulders are mobile as they bend and extend to lower the long spine to the floor.

2) Egg Stretch #2

Pull back into an egg shape, sitz bones resting on the heels, forehead to the floor. For this variation, reach the arms out along the floor over the head to stretch out the chest. Reach the sitz bones away from the top of the head, lengthening the lumbar spine, and breathe into the sides and back of the rib cage.

IMAGERY

For *Egg Stretch #2*, see the whole body breathing and expanding, air filling the ribs, pelvis, and lumbar area. Imagine the scapulae heavy and weighted, sliding around the rib cage towards the floor. Imagine the arms getting longer on each exhale, and the chest widening and expanding.

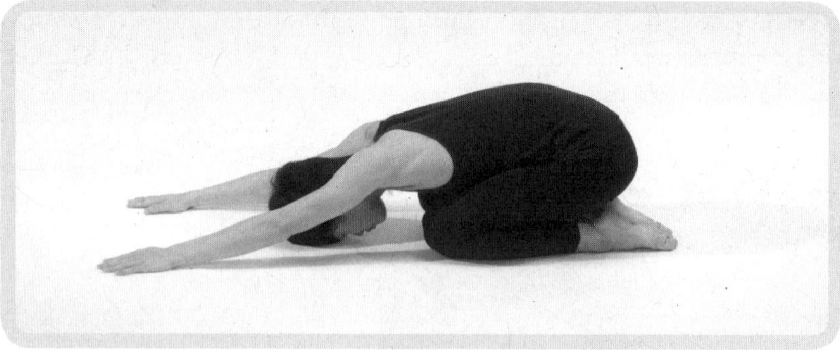

3) Shoulder Rolls

From the *Egg Stretch #2*, roll the torso up so that the body is upright, sitting on the heels. In a slow and continuous motion, on counts 1,2,3, circle the right shoulder in a front to back direction; that is, taking the shoulder forward, up, back, and down; on 2,2,3, repeat left, and continue alternating the shoulders until eight total circles have been completed (8-3s of music, see photo 1). Now reverse the direction, and do eight circles alternating sides moving back to front. Slowing to half time, do four circles of both shoulders front to back (8-3s of music, or 2-3s for each circle, see photos 2–4). Reverse the direction, and do four circles of both shoulders moving back to front (8-3s of music, or 2-3s for each circle). Finally, do a full arm circle with the right arm front to back; the palm should face in towards the midline of the body at the start of the circle, and then at the top of the movement as the hand reaches to the ceiling, the palm should slowly rotate to face out away from the body and eventually down to the floor behind the body (see photo 5). Repeat left, and alternate four times (8-3s of music, or 2-3s for each circle). As an added neck stretch, the head can rotate away from the arm as the arm is reaching back behind the body (see photo 6).

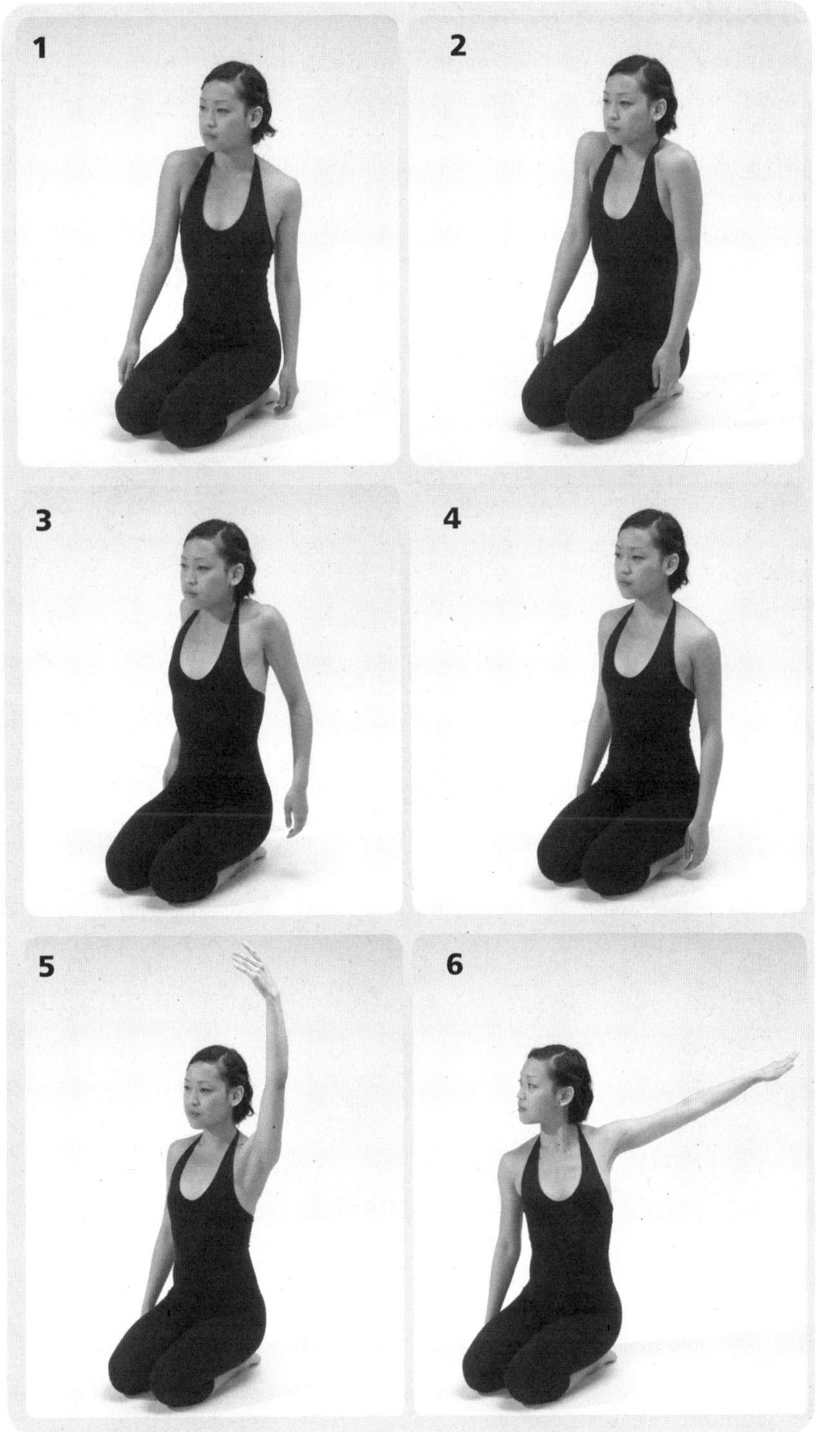

IMAGERY

For *Shoulder Rolls*, imagine that the upper body is in water, and the action of the shoulders circling is like swimming. For the final arm circles, imagine the hands reaching out far from the shoulders and extending into the space, drawing large ovals on either side of the body.

4) Final Stretches

The following stretches can be done for the first time at this point in the session, or repeated here if they were done in Part Three – Flexibility Series:

Hip Flexor Lunge (page 80)

Mountain (page 82)

Standing and Hanging (page 82)

IMAGERY

For *Final Stretches*, refer to the images in Part Three – Flexibility Series.

5) Rolling Up to Stance

At the end of *Standing and Hanging*, from a demi plié, close the eyes, and roll up to stance with the legs parallel and the arms relaxed at the sides of the body. This rolling action should be done sequentially. First, drop the pelvis to neutral alignment (pubic bone and tailbone level to the floor), maintaining the plié. Next, float the rib cage up above the pelvis, and slide the shoulder blades wide into the space. Finally, float the neck and head up above the rib cage to finish. Note: As the spine is rolling up to vertical, lengthen through the legs so that the legs are fully extended by the time the body is upright. Throughout this rolling action, the feet are in parallel, and the width of the hip sockets.

IMAGERY

For *Rolling Up to Stance*, imagine energy coming up from the floor through the bottoms of the feet, rising up the legs, and filling the pelvis. As the spine is rolling up, see the energy climbing up the spine, filling the rib cage, and finally flowing up the neck and into the head. See the line of energy going out the top of the head into the space above the body.

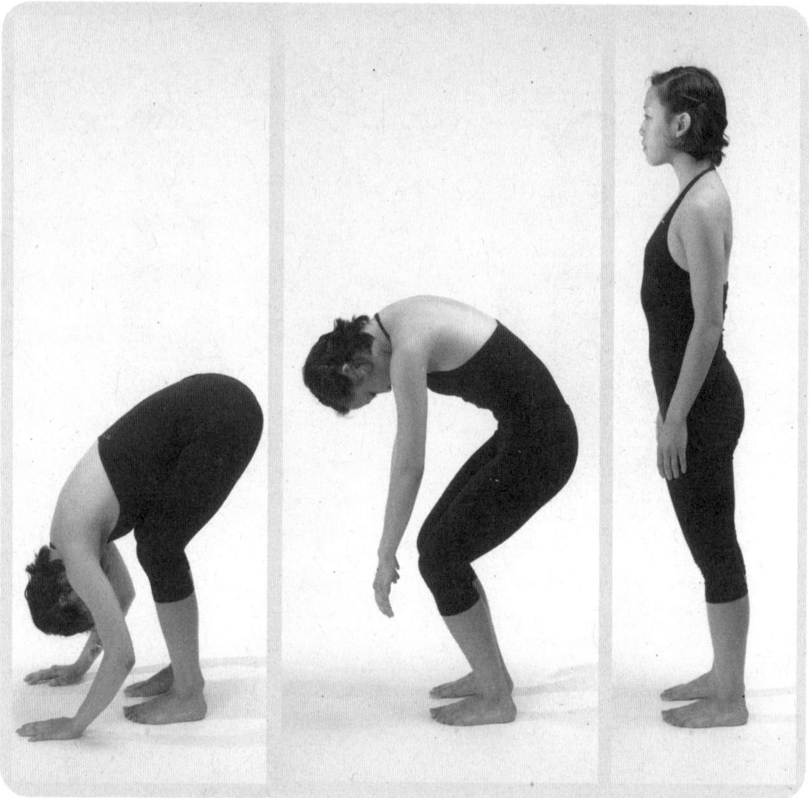

6) Balancing Work

There are many possible variations to assist in developing proprioception for improved balance. Each of the balances in this section can be attempted for ten to thirty seconds.

Variation 1 – With eyes closed, slowly relevé in parallel. If this is very difficult for the dancers, begin by taking the heels just off of the floor. When balancing on the balls of the feet becomes easier, the dancers can attempt the full rise.

Variation 2 – With the weight on both feet (not on relevé) and the eyes closed, shift the weight over to the right foot. Bend the left knee and lift the left foot off the floor; point the foot and place it at the side of the right ankle. Return to two feet and repeat on the other side.

Variation 3 – Demi plié on both feet, and do the same shift to one foot as in Variation 2. While on the right foot in plié, slowly straighten the right foot. Return to two feet and repeat on the other side.

Variation 4 – Reverse the actions of Variations 2 and 3 so that first the weight is shifted to one foot, and then demi plié. In the demi plié, return to two feet, and straighten the legs.

Variation 5 – Repeat Variation 2, and while supporting the weight on one foot, bring the left foot to the side of the right knee. Return to two feet and repeat on the other side.

Variation 6 – Start balanced on the right foot, with the left foot pointed at the ankle. On count 1, take a large step forward onto the left foot, and hold count 2. Repeat the step onto the right foot 3, hold 4, step side left 5, hold 6, side step right 7, hold 8. Repeat, going to the back and to the side for another eight counts. These steps can also be done onto a plié on the supporting leg. Finally, any of the balances described can be done with the legs turned out instead of parallel. Arm gestures can be added to any of the balances as well, moving the arms to the oval in front of the ribs, to second position or to fifth position. The tempo of these movements can begin very slowly, eventually accelerating. All of these variations increase the challenges to the balancing mechanisms.

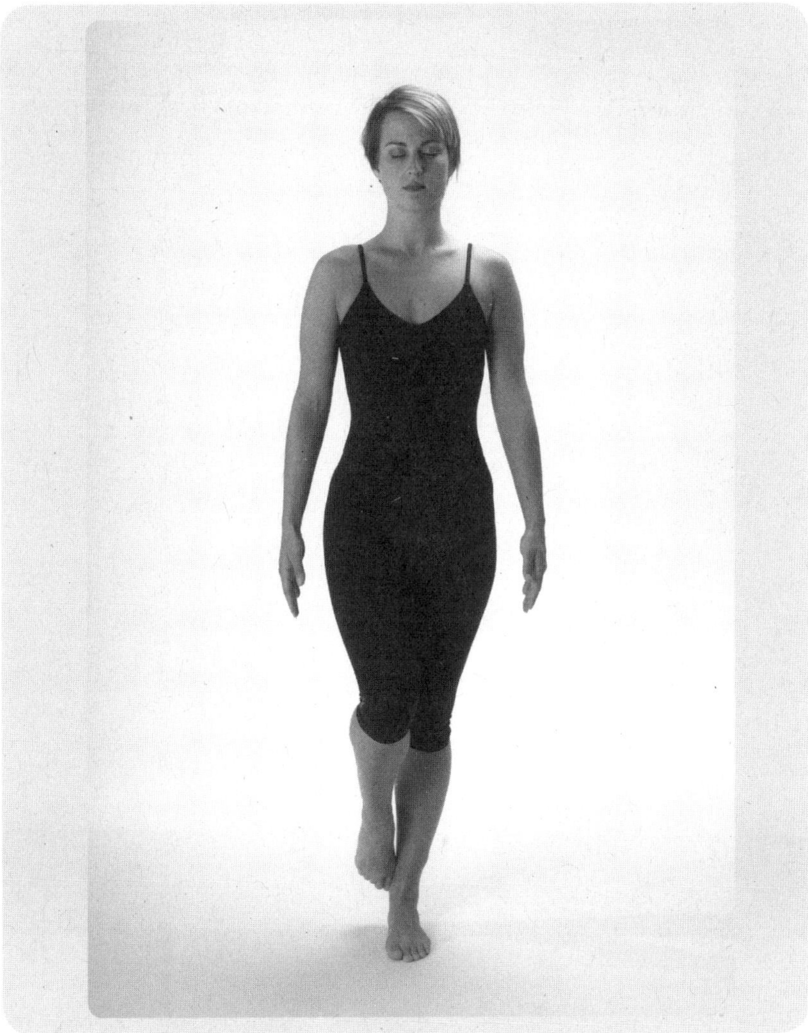

IMAGERY

For *Balancing Work*, visualize the plumb line through the body; when seeing the body from the side, it falls through the centre of the head and ears, the rib cage, the pelvis, the greater trochanters of the femurs (when in parallel position), just behind the centre of the knee joint, and just in front of the malleoli (ankle bones) before diving into the floor. Seeing the body from the front or back, the plumb line divides the body into equal right and left sides. See this plumb line as a strong energetic line or cord deep in the centre of the body, while the surfaces of the body soften and melt. For all of the balances, this line of energy should reach up and out of the top of the head, and down into the floor from the bottoms of the feet. As the weight shifts to one foot (e.g., in Variation 2), imagine that the navel lines up over the supporting foot and the hip bones stay in a line parallel to the floor, so that the pelvis translates sideways, and does not tilt or twist to shift the weight. Imagine the body as a volcano, with the hot lava rising up from the floor deep in the centre of the body, into the feet and through the pelvis and spine, shooting out of the top of the head, and pouring down the surfaces on all sides of the body.

Notes for Teachers

For *Push-Ups*, the dancers can use the variation with the weight on the knees if the full push-up as described above is too difficult. For dancers with very weak upper limbs and/or core support, this exercise can be started in stance position using a wall, gradually moving the feet further away from the wall. For dancers who desire a greater challenge, the feet can be elevated on a step, or an exercise ball can be used under the ankles.

For *Shoulder Rolls*, if sitting on the heels is painful to the knees or the ankles, or for dancers with knee problems of any kind, sit crossed-legged for this exercise instead of sitting back on the heels. Remind the dancers to keep the top of the head and spine lengthening up towards the ceiling throughout the circles.

For *Rolling Up to Stance* and *Balancing Work*, verbal cues and imagery from the teacher will depend on the specific imbalances and weaknesses each dancer is attempting to correct. No one image will work for an entire group. The teacher can provide many images and suggestions, and allow the dancers to experiment and explore. In the end, each dancer should be encouraged to develop his or her own series of images and to become familiar with the sensory input of good muscle balance to use for this work, and to transfer to the dance class and rehearsal.

Review Questions

Introduction

1. List several goals of a good conditioning program for dancers.
2. Define the following conditioning terms: muscular strength and endurance; flexibility and range of motion; frequency, duration and intensity; proprioception; and neural recruitment.
3. What are the five principles of C-I Training? Describe each principle and why each one is important.
4. Define imagery, and name some of the early somatic pioneers.
5. Why is imagery combined with conditioning in C-I Training?
6. What is transfer of training? Give some examples.

Part One: Fundamental Principles and Warm-Up

1. Define neutral pelvis and describe one exercise that can assist in understanding how to find and maintain a neutral pelvis.
2. What is core initiation? Describe the exercise called *The Big X*.
3. What is the purpose of *Rock and Stir*?
4. Name two areas of weakness that are common in the muscles of the feet and ankles of dancers, and describe two exercises that address these areas.
5. Describe movements of the scapulae that are common in every day life but inhibited in dance gestures. Explain two images that can assist the dancer in this movement patterning.
6. Define narrowing and hollowing. Describe the exercises called *Undercurves and Overcurves*. Give four images described in this book, and create two of your own that assist in these exercises.
7. Describe four purposes of the exercise called *The Clock*, and name one postural problem that this exercise can address.
8. What is the purpose of ankle circles?
9. What images would you use doing the exercise *Extending the Legs with Turnout*, and how would you apply these to standing work?

Part Two: Legwork and Core Support

1. What are the three central goals of the section called "Legwork and Core Support?"
2. Describe turnout, and how the exercises called *Rotating In and Out* and *Lowering and Raising the Leg* address the alignment of the hip, knee, ankle and foot for standing work.
3. What is the purpose of the exercises *Touch Reach Series* and *Plié Reach Series*? How are they different?

4. Describe the two variations of the *Exercise on 6 for the Spine*, and give five images that assist in executing these exercises correctly.
5. What is the purpose of the *Jiggles*? Why are there two directions?
6. How would an exercise designed to increase flexibility (*Second Position Extensions on 3*) inform the dancer about correct placement of the legs and spine in standing work?

Part Three: Flexibility Series

1. Name five reasons to encourage flexibility in dancers.
2. Describe images for the exercise called *Sitting with Folded Legs with Variations*.
3. What is the purpose of the exercise *Hanging over Extended Legs*, and how might this exercise improve the dancer's technique?
4. Describe images for the exercise called *Pretzel*. What might these images achieve in this exercise?
5. What is the purpose of the exercises called *Quadriceps Variations*, and what common problems in dancers do these exercises address?
6. What is the purpose of the exercise called *Hip Flexor Lunge*? Name some dance movements that can be improved by doing this exercise.
7. Describe images for the exercise called *Mountain*.

Part Four: Développé and Rond de Jambe Series

1. Name four purposes or goals of the section called "Développé and Rond de Jambe Series." How does the approach and execution of this material support these underlying goals?
2. Describe the starting position for the "Développé and Rond de Jambe Series." How would you best describe the spine? How would you organize the feet? Are you attempting to get the knees on the floor? Are you actively engaged in the core at the start?
3. Why is adding the rond de jambe much more difficult than the simple développé?
4. Images for the "Développé and Rond de Jambe Series" accommodate both increased range and increased stability. Describe some of these images. Is increasing range of motion or increasing stability more important for you personally as a dancer? Can you invent your own images to assist you in achieving this goal?

Part Five: Developing Turnout

1. Name and describe the four goals of the section called "Developing Turnout."

2. Describe the purposes of the exercises called *Clams*. Why are the later versions (*Full Clam* and *Beyond the Clam*) not recommended for beginners?
3. Describe two images for *Clams*, and the specific purpose of each image.
4. What general purpose do the three exercises called *Leg Lifts for the Outer Leg*, *Pressing to the Back*, and *Legs Lifts for the Inner Leg* accomplish? Name the specific purpose (target muscle group) for each of these exercises.
5. Describe the three component parts to the group of exercises called *Dancing Legs (for Advanced Dancers)*. Describe three images the dancer can use for this series.
6. Why is there a need to do a spiral stretch at end of all of the side lying exercises in "Developing Turnout?"
7. Describe the starting position for *Beats*. What is meant by "the bowl of the body"? Give one image for the leg action during *Beats*.

Part Six: On Extension

1. What are five general goals of the section called "On Extension?"
2. What are three specific goals of *Massaging the Heart*?
3. What correction do dancers often receive about their shoulders, and how can *Shrugs – Descending Scapulae* address this issue? What image might you use doing this exercise that can be applied to standing and traveling work?
4. Name four specific goals of the section called "Legwork in Extension."
5. Describe two images for *Double Leg Extensions*, and the purpose of each image.
6. Describe two variations of *Alternating Leg Lifts*, and what each variation addresses. How are the arms used differently in the two variations?
7. In what ways are *Beats in Low Arabesque* different from *Beats* in the section "A Trip Around the Hip?" Why might dancers want to do both?
8. Describe the four variations of "The Ferris Wheel: Spine in Extension." Name one distinct purpose of each variation.

Part Seven: Final Strength and Stretch

1. Why would dancers choose to incorporate *Push-Ups* into their conditioning? Can you name a movement you might do in choreography or class that would require what push-ups provide?
2. What is the purpose of the two egg stretches?

3. Describe images you might use doing *Shoulder Rolls*, and what these images might achieve. Can you invent your own images for this exercise?
4. What is the difference in doing stretches in the middle of C-I Training versus at the end in "Final Strength and Stretch?"
5. What is the importance of *Rolling Up to Stance*, and how would you describe this process in your own words?
6. Why would one choose to perform balances with the eyes closed? Describe some images that might assist in making balance easier in this condition.

Postural Problems and Muscle Imbalances

This section is to address postural problems and muscle imbalances (strength and stretch) that are commonly seen in dancers. These exercises can assist in providing the strength and flexibility/release needed in specific muscle groups. With guidance and insight from the teacher, the dancer can learn to align the body and use the muscles more efficiently. While this work is not rehabilitation for injuries, it is believed that a better-aligned, balanced body will be less predisposed to injury. For injuries or chronic pain, it is important to seek medical advice.

Pectoralis Minor Syndrome (rounded shoulders)

Part	Letter	Ex. #	Exercise Name	Pg #
One	B	2	Rocking the Boat – Angels in the Snow	8
One	C	1	Stretch Out	9
One	G	2	The Clock	31
One	G	3	The First Spiral Stretch	32
One	G	4	The Second Spiral Stretch	32
Seven	N/A	3	Shoulder Rolls	130

Elevated Scapulae (raised shoulders)

Part	Letter	Ex. #	Exercise Name	Pg #
One	B	2	Rocking the Boat – Angels in the Snow	8
Three	N/A	5	Sitting in Second Position (A & C)	76
Six	A	3	Shrugs – Descending Scapulae	113
Six	A	4	Port de Bras	114

Winged Scapulae (also do exercises for Pectoralis minor syndrome)

Part	Letter	Ex. #	Exercise Name	Pg #
One	E	1	Arm Series on 8	19
Six	A	2	Massaging the Heart – Retreating and Advancing the Sternum	112
Seven	N/A	1	Push-ups (particularly Scapular Push-ups with Plank variation)	128

Tight (immobile) Thoracic Spine

Part	Letter	Ex. #	Exercise Name	Pg #
One	G	2	The Clock	31
Six	A	1	Sphinx	112
Six	A	2	Massaging the Heart – Retreating and Advancing the Sternum	112
Six	C	1	Chest Lifts on 3s Plain	124
Six	C	2	Flying Bird – Chest Lifts on 3s with Arms Behind	125
Six	C	3	Widening the Back – Chest Lifts on 3s with Arms in Second	125
Six	C	4	Final Strength Work – Chest Lifts on 3s with Arms in Fifth	126
Six	C	5	Final Rest – Egg Stretch	126

Weak Abdominals and Poor Core Support (possibly swayback)

Part	Letter	Ex. #	Exercise Name	Pg #
One	B	1	The Big X – Core Initiation	7
One	F	1	Narrowing and Hollowing	24
One	F	2	Undercurves	25
One	F	3	Undercurves and Overcurves	26
One	F	4	Preparations for Small Curls	26
One	F	5	Small Curls	27
One	F	6	Small Curls with a Twist	28
One	F	7	Advanced Variation	28
Two	A	4	Core Support with Moving Legs – Variation 1: Touch Reach Series	52
Two	A	4	Core Support with Moving Legs – Variation 2: Plié Reach Series	54
Two	B	1	Exercise on 6 for the Spine – Variation 1: Roll-Down	60
Two	B	1	Exercise on 6 for the Spine – Variation 2: Arch Down	62
Two	B	2	Extensions from the Bridge	63
Five	A	2	Full Clam	98
Five	A	3	Beyond the Clam – Variation 1: Rotations on a Slow 4	99
Five	A	3	Beyond the Clam – Variation 2: Pulses on a Fast 3/8	100
Five	B	6	Beats	108
Six	A	2	Massaging the Heart – Retreating and Advancing the Sternum	112
Seven	N/A	1	Push-Ups	128

Tight Hip Flexors (assist with psoas tendon problems, swayback)

Part	Letter	Ex. #	Exercise Name	Pg #
One	F	2	Undercurves	25
One	F	3	Undercurves and Overcurves	26
Two	B	1	Exercise on 6 for the Spine – Variation 1: Roll-Down	60
Two	B	1	Exercise on 6 for the Spine – Variation 2: Arch Down	62
Two	B	2	Extensions from the Bridge	63
Three	N/A	7	Hip Flexor Lunge	80
Five	B	2	Pressing to the Back	104
Six	B	1	Double Leg Extension	117
Six	B	2	Parallel Alternating Leg Lifts	117

Tight Hamstrings (especially lateral)

Part	Letter	Ex. #	Exercise Name	Pg #
Two	A	2	Lowering and Raising the Leg	50
Two	A	3	Flexibility Series – (A) Hamstrings	50
Two	A	3	Flexibility Series – (B) Hamstrings with leg across	51
Three	N/A	3	Hanging over Extended Legs	74
Three	N/A	9	Standing and Hanging	82

Weak Hamstrings

Part	Letter	Ex. #	Exercise Name	Pg #
Two	B	1	Exercise on 6 for the Spine – Variation 1: Roll-Down	60
Two	B	1	Exercise on 6 for the Spine – Variation 2: Arch Down	62
Two	B	2	Extensions from the Bridge	63
Five	B	2	Pressing to the Back	104
Six	B	1	Double Leg Extension	117
Six	B	2	Parallel Alternating Leg Lifts	117
Six	B	3	Turned Out Alternating Leg Lifts	118
Six	B	3	Turned Out Alternating Leg Lifts – Variation 1: Flexing the Foot	119
Six	B	3	Turned Out Alternating Leg Lifts – Variation 2: Bending the Knee	119
Six	B	4	Exercise on 6 for the Arabesque	120
Six	B	5	Beats in Low Arabesque	122

Weak (underused) Adductors (inner thighs)

Part	Letter	Ex. #	Exercise Name	Pg #
One	I	4	Extending the Legs with Turnout	40
Two	B	1	Exercise on 6 for the Spine – Variation 1: Roll-Down	60
Two	B	1	Exercise on 6 for the Spine – Variation 2: Arch Down	62
Two	B	2	Extensions from the Bridge	63
Five	B	3	Leg Lifts for the Inner Leg	104
Five	B	6	Beats	108
Six	B	5	Beats in Low Arabesque	122

Tight Outward Rotators (especially the deep rotators)

Part	Letter	Ex. #	Exercise Name	Pg #
One	G	3	The First Spiral Stretch	32
One	G	4	The Second Spiral Stretch	32
Two	A	3	Flexibility Series – (C) Over-Crossed Passé	51
Two	A	3	Flexibility Series – (D) Attitude Across	52
Three	N/A	1	Sitting with Folded Legs (with Variations)	72
Three	N/A	4	Pretzel	75
Three	N/A	7	Hip Flexor Lunge – Variation B	80

Weak Inward Rotators/Abductors (outer hips)

Part	Letter	Ex. #	Exercise Name	Pg #
Two	A	1	Rotating In and Out	44
Two	B	1	Exercise on 6 for the Spine – Variation 1: Roll-Down	60
Two	B	1	Exercise on 6 for the Spine – Variation 2: Arch Down	62
Two	B	2	Extensions from the Bridge	63
Five	B	1	Leg Lifts for the Outer Leg	102
Six	B	1	Double Leg Extensions	117
Six	B	2	Parallel Alternating Leg Lifts	117

Tight quadriceps / IT band

Part	Letter	Ex. #	Exercise Name	Pg #
Three	N/A	6	Quadriceps Variations	78
Three	N/A	7	Hip Flexor Lunge – Variation B	80

Lateral and Medial Vastus Imbalance (outer quad tighter than inner quad, inner legs weak and underused)

Part	Letter	Ex. #	Exercise Name	Pg #
Two	A	4	Core Support with Moving Legs – Variation 1: Touch Reach Series	52
Two	B	1	Exercise on 6 for the Spine – Variation 1: Roll-Down	60
Two	B	1	Exercise on 6 for the Spine – Variation 2: Arch Down	62
Two	B	2	Extensions from the Bridge	63
Three	N/A	7	Hip Flexor Lunge – Variation B	80

Hyperextended Knees

Part	Letter	Ex. #	Exercise Name	Pg #
One	I	4	Extending the Legs with Turnout	40
Two	A	4	Core Support with Moving Legs – Variation 2: Plié Reach Series	54
Six	B	1	Double Leg Extensions	117
Six	B	5	Beats in Low Arabesque	122

Weak Dorsiflexors (front of the shin)

Part	Letter	Ex. #	Exercise Name	Pg #
One	D	1	Points and Squeezy Flexes	12

Tight Calves

Part	Letter	Ex. #	Exercise Name	Pg #
Three	N/A	3	Handing Over Extended Legs (b)	74
Three	N/A	8	Mountain	82
Three	N/A	9	Standing and Hanging	82

Pronated Feet (rolling in) and Supinated Feet (rolling out, especially in relevé)

Part	Letter	Ex. #	Exercise Name	Pg #
One	D	1	Points and Squeezy Flexes	12
One	D	2	U-Shapes for the Ankles	15
Two	A	1	Rotating In and Out: Variations	46, 48

Weak Arches

Part	Letter	Ex. #	Exercise Name	Pg #
One	D	1	Points and Squeezy Flexes	12
One	D	2	U-Shapes for the Ankles	15

Anterior view of the human skeleton.

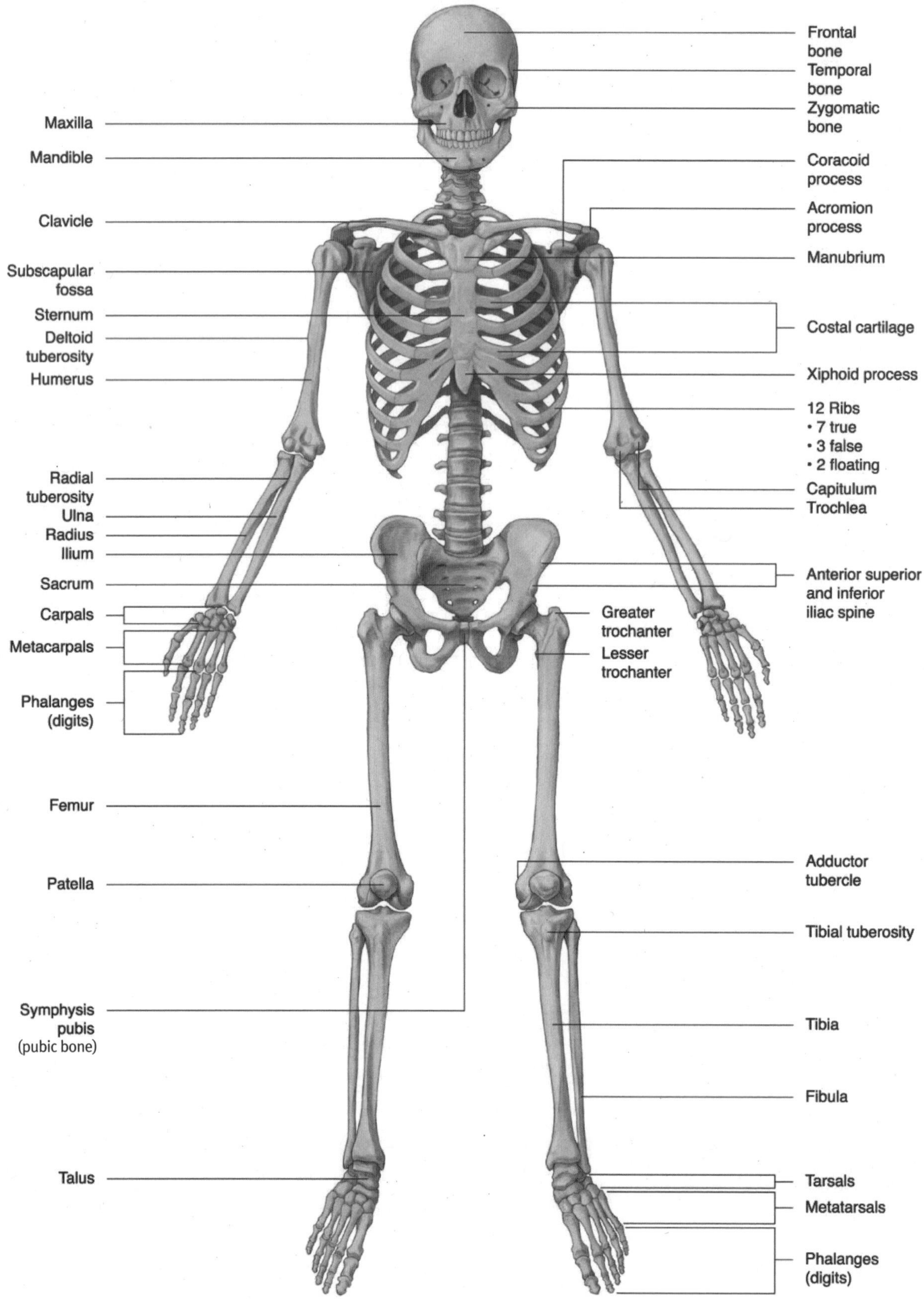

Posterior view of the human skeleton.

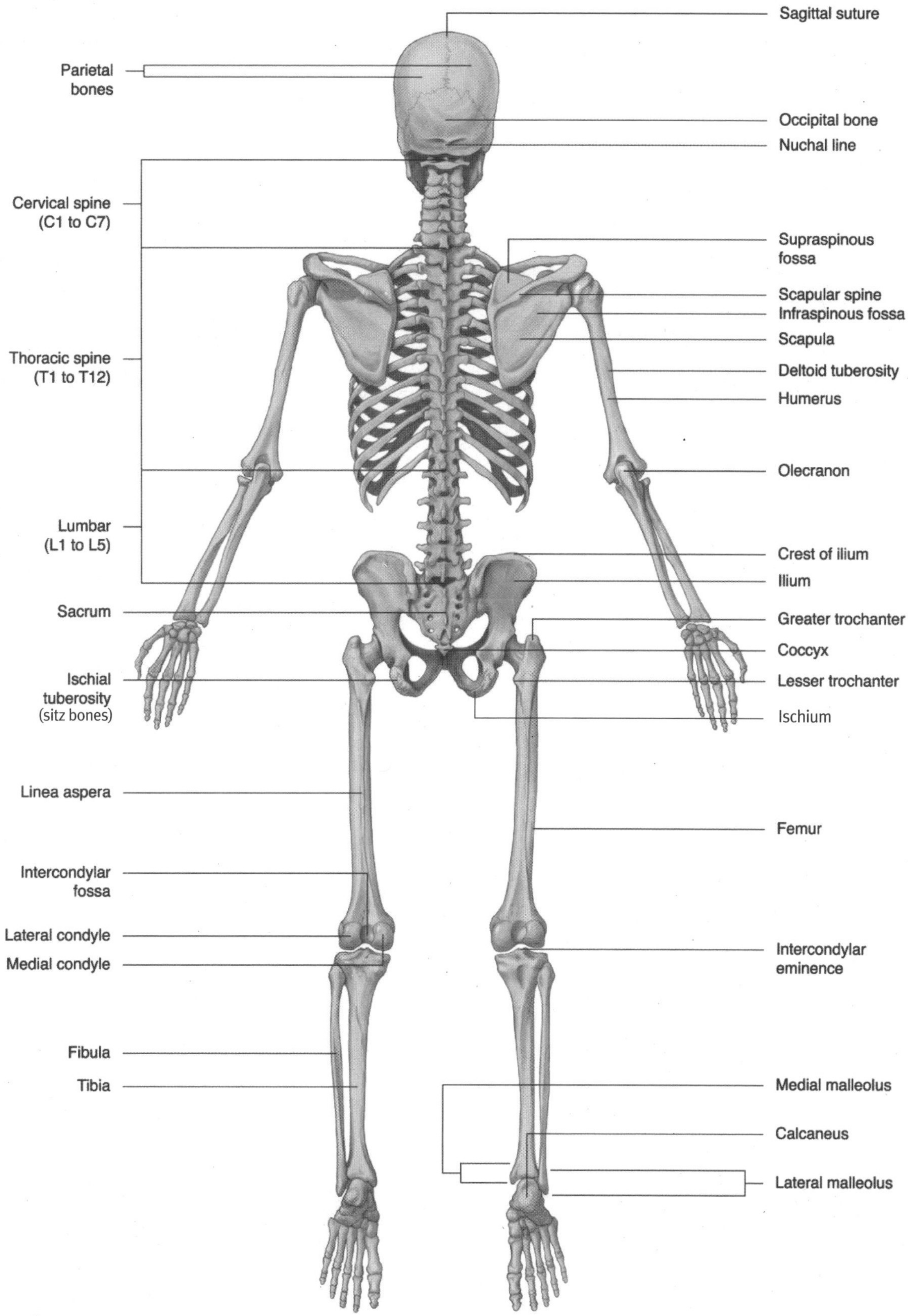

Anterior view of the muscular system.

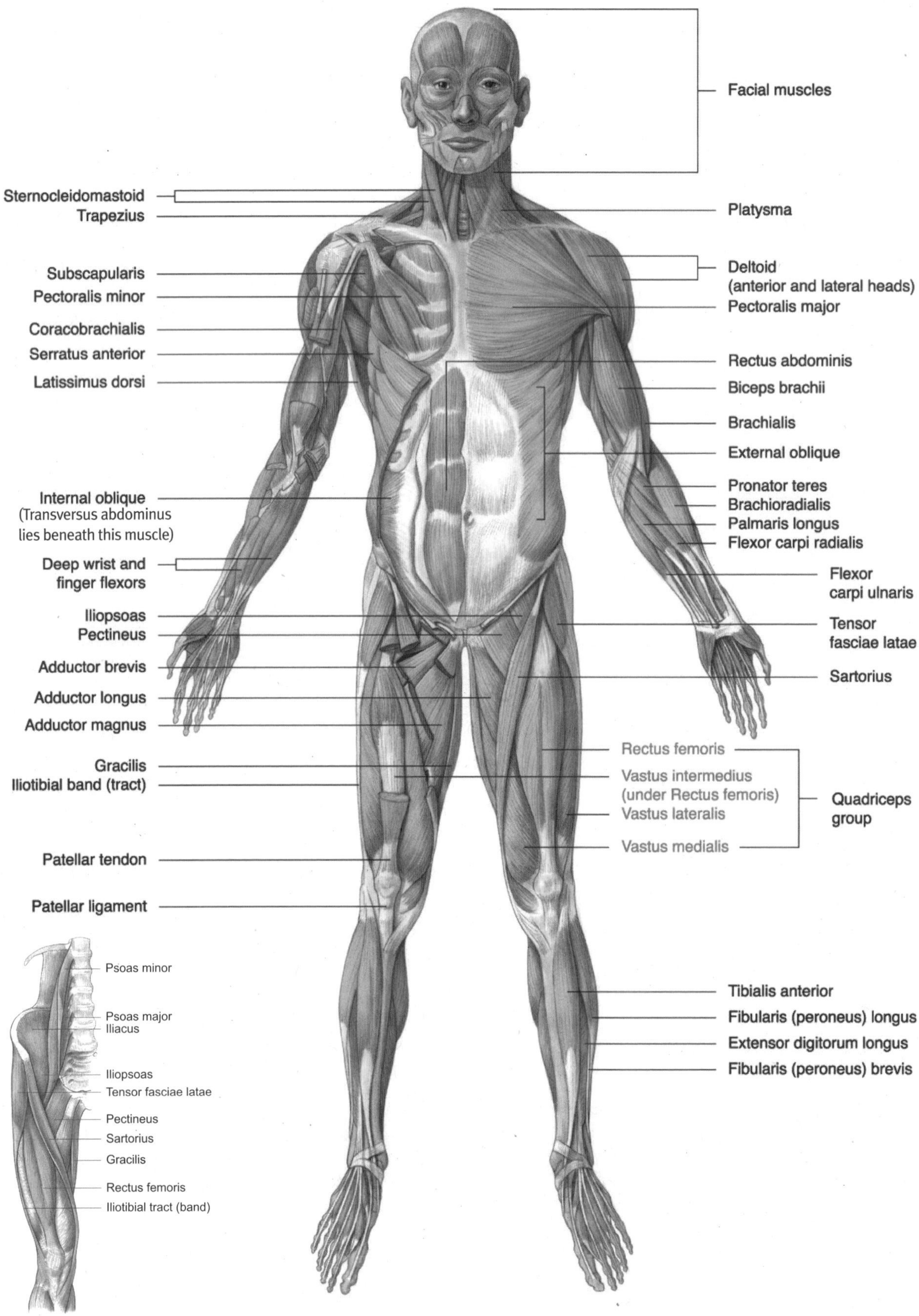

Posterior view of the muscular system.

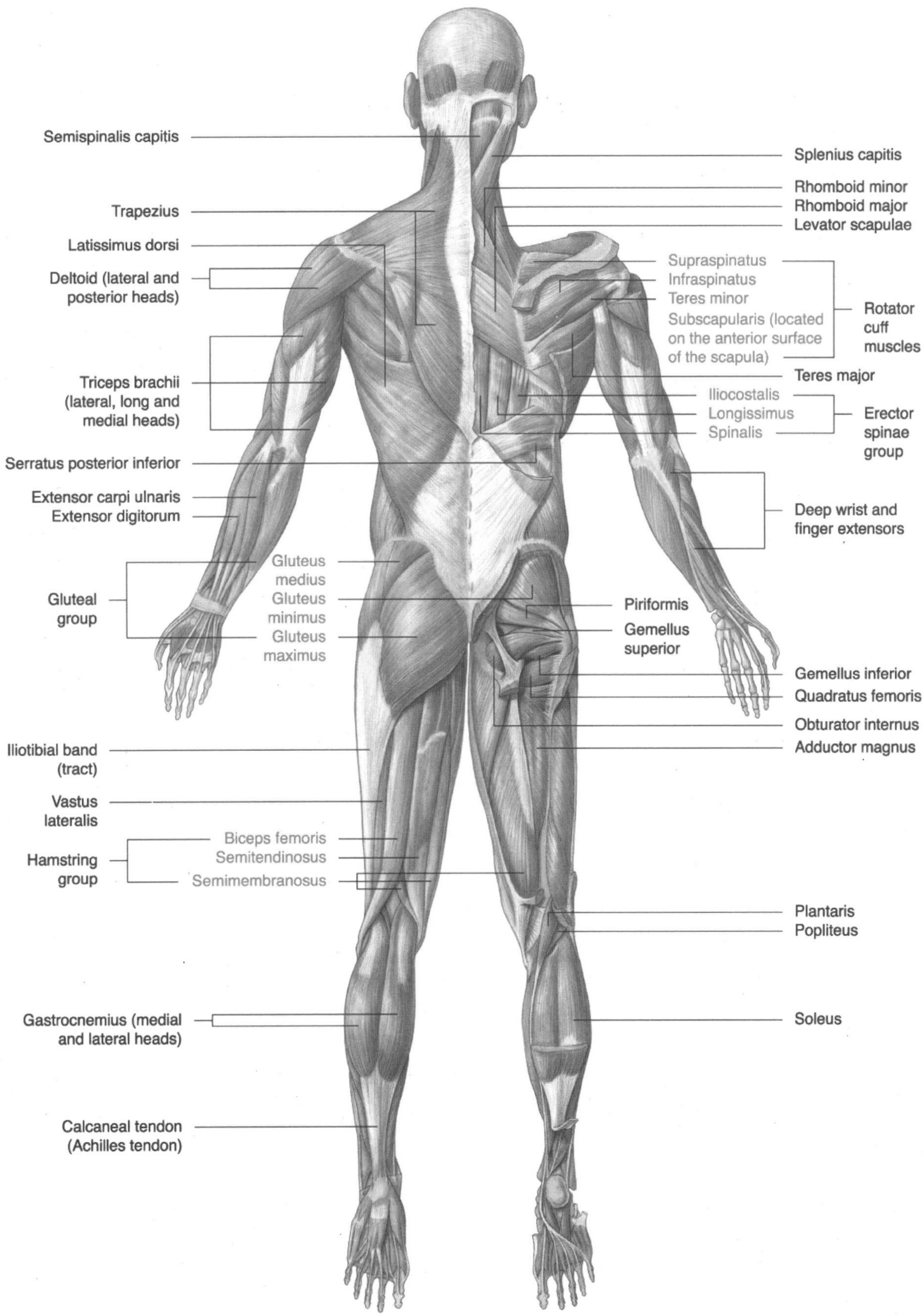

Appendix of Terminology

Planes of Movement

Sagittal: The vertical plane that divides the body into right and left sides, sometimes called the "Wheel Plane."

Frontal or Coronal: The vertical plane that divides the body into front and back portions, sometimes called the "Door Plane."

Transverse or Horizontal: The horizontal plane that divides the body into upper and lower portions, sometimes called the "Table Plane."

Movement Terms

Flexion: The decrease in the angle of two articulating bones in the sagittal plane. Example: From standing position, lifting one leg to a parallel passé. This involves flexion of both the hip and the knee joints. Curving forward is flexion of the spine.

Extension: The increase in the angle of two articulating bones in the sagittal plane. The return to neutral from the flexed position. Example: Bringing the leg from parallel passé back to standing position.

Hyperextension: Continuation of extension beyond anatomical neutral. Example: Arabesque involves hyperextension of the hip and the low back, which arches to achieve the full range of motion.

Abduction: The movement of a bone in the frontal plane away from the midline of the body. Example: Lifting the arms out to second position.

Adduction: The movement of a bone in the frontal plane towards from the midline of the body. Example: Lowering the arms from second position to straight down.

Outward rotation: Also called lateral or external rotation, the movement of a bone around its own axis, away from the midline of the body. Example: Both the hip joint and the shoulder outward rotate. Standing in classical first is a position of outward rotation.

Inward rotation: Also called medial or internal rotation, the movement of a bone around its own axis, towards the midline of the body. Example: Both the hip joint and the shoulder inward rotate.

Supination: This movement term is used for both the forearm (radio-ulnar joint) and for the foot. Movement of the forearm in which the palm is turned anteriorly (or away from the midline of the body). When standing, supination occurs as the foot rolls outwards, placing most of the weight onto the outside of the foot and raising the arch. Supination combines inversion (moving the soles of the feet medially) and adduction of the foot. Example: When the foot is "sickled," it is supinated.

Pronation: This movement term is used for both the forearm (radio-ulnar joint) and the foot. Movement of the forearm in which the palm is turned posteriorly, or towards the midline of the body. When standing, pronation occurs as the foot rolls inward, placing most of the weight onto the inside of the foot and lowering the arch. Pronation combines eversion (moving the soles of the feet laterally) and abduction of the foot. Example: When the foot is "winged," it is pronated.

Horizontal flexion: This movement of the arm starts from the abducted position of the shoulder joint. Movement of the arm forward in the transverse plane. Example: Moving the arm from second position to first arabesque.

Horizontal extension: Movement of the arm backwards in the transverse plane. Example: Moving the arm from first arabesque out to second position.

Elevation: Upward movement of the scapulae (shoulder blades). Example: Shrugging the shoulders.

Depression: Downward movement of the scapulae (shoulder blades). Example: Dropping the shoulders back to neutral.

Upward rotation: Rotary movement of the scapulae; moving inferior angle (bottom) of scapulae laterally and upward. Example: This movement of the scapulae only occurs when the arms are lifting. The scapulae revolve to allow for greater range of motion in the arm, such as from second position to fifth position.

Downward rotation: Rotary movement of the scapulae; moving inferior angle (bottom) of scapulae medially and downward. Example: The return of the scapulae as the arms move from fifth position to second position and back down to neutral.

Protraction: Moving the scapulae away from the spine and towards the front of the rib cage. This movement is sometimes called abduction of the scapulae because it is movement away from the body's midline. Example: Rounding the shoulders forward.

Retraction: Moving the scapulae towards the spine and away from the front of the rib cage; that is, returning to neutral from the protracted position. This movement is sometimes called adduction of the scapulae because it is movement away from the body's midline. Example: Moving the shoulders from a rounded position to an open, wide position.

Plantar flexion: Bending at the ankle joint in the sagittal plane, so that the toes move away from the front of the shin bone. Example: Dancers call this "pointing the foot." Relevé is also an example of plantar flexion.

Dorsiflexion: Bending at the ankle joint in the sagittal plane, so that the toes move towards the front of the shin bone. Example: Dancers call this "flexing the foot." When the dancer pliés, dorsiflexion at the ankle increases.

Lateral flexion: A movement of the spine in the frontal plane to the left or to the right. Example: Side-bending.

Rotation left and right: Turning of the spine on its vertical axis. Example: Turning or spiraling the spine. Spotting requires fast rotation of the cervical spine.

Circumduction: Range of movements that create a complete circle; it occurs as a result of a continuous sequence of flexion, abduction, extension, and adduction. Example: Rond de jambe.

Types of Muscle Contraction

A contraction is called **concentric** when the muscle is working but shortening in length, such as when one is lifting one's leg.

A contraction is called **eccentric** when the muscle is working but lengthening. For a muscle to be working and lengthening, there must be an outside force that exceeds the force of the muscle, such as the pull of gravity when slowly lowering one's leg.

A contraction is called **isometric** when the muscle is working but no change in length is occurring. There must be an opposing force, such as holding the leg in one place against the force of gravity.

Additional Terms

Lying **supine** means lying on one's back with the front of the body facing the ceiling. Lying prone means lying on one's front with the back of the body facing the ceiling.

Proximal refers to being nearer to the origin or midline of the body. **Distal** refers to being further from the origin or midline of the body. For example, the head of the femur (thigh bone) is proximal while the end of the femur at the knee is distal.

Bibliography

Alexander, F. M. *The Use of the Self.* Long Beach, CA: Centerline Press, 1985.

Alter, M. *Science of Flexibility* (3rd ed.). Champaign, IL: Human Kinetics Publishers, Inc., 2004.

Arnheim, D. *Dance Injuries: Their Prevention and Care* (3rd ed.). Princeton, NJ: Princeton Book Company, 1991.

Barnes, M. A., D. Krasnow, S.J. Tupling, and M. Thomas. Knee rotation in classical dancers during the grand plié. *Medical Problems of Performing Artists*, 15, 140–7, 2000.

Bartenieff, I., with D. Lewis. *Body movement: Coping with the environment.* New York: Gordon and Breach, Science Publishers, 1980.

Basmajian, J.V. *Primary Anatomy* (8th ed.). Baltimore, MD: Williams and Wilkens, 1982.

Batson, G. Conscious use of the human body in movement: The peripheral neuroanatomic basis of the Alexander Technique. *Medical Problems of Performing Artists*, 11(1), 3–11, 1996.

Calais-Germain, B. *Anatomy of Movement.* Seattle, WA: Eastland Press, 1991.

Chatfield, S. J., D. H. Krasnow, A. Herman, and G. Blessing. A descriptive analysis of kinematic and electromyographic relationships of the core during forward stepping in beginning and expert dancers. *Journal of Dance Medicine & Science*, 11/3, 76–84, 2007.

Clarkson, P. M., and M. Skrinar. *Science of Dance Training.* Champaign, IL: Human Kinetics Books, 1988.

Clippinger, K. *Dance Anatomy and Kinesiology.* Champaign, IL: Human Kinetics, 2006.

Dowd, I. *Taking Root to Fly* (2nd ed.). North Hampton, MA: Contact Collaborations, 1990.

Feldenkrais, M. *Awareness Through Movement: Health Exercises for Personal Growth.* New York: Harper & Row Publishers, 1972.

Fitt, S. S. *Dance Kinesiology* (2nd ed.). New York: Schirmer Books, 1996.

Franklin, E. *Dynamic Alignment through Imagery.* Champaign, IL: Human Kinetics, 1996.

Franklin, E. *Dance Imagery for Technique and Performance.* Champaign, IL: Human Kinetics, 1996.

Friedman, P., and G. Eisen. *The Pilates Method of Physical and Mental Conditioning.* Garden City, NY: Doubleday and Company, 1980.

Gray, H. *Gray's Anatomy* (15th ed.). New York: Bounty Books, 1977.

Grossman, G., D. Krasnow, and T. M. Welsh. Effective use of turnout: Biomechanical, neuromuscular, and behavioral considerations. *Journal of Dance Education*, 5/1, 15–27, 2005.

Haas, J. G. *Dance Anatomy*. Champaign, IL: Human Kinetics, 2010.

Hackney, P. Remembering Irmgard. *Contact Quarterly*, 18(1), 13-20, 1993.

Hamilton, N., W. Weimar, and K. Luttgens. *Kinesiology: Scientific Basis of Human Motion* (11th ed.). Boston, MA: McGraw-Hill, 2008.

Haywood, K. M., and N. Getchell. *Life Span Motor Development* (4th ed.). Champaign, IL: Human Kinetics, 2005.

Kandel, E. R., J. H. Schwartz, and T. M. Jessell. (Eds.). *Principles of Neural Science* (3rd ed.). New York: Elsevier Science Publishing Company, 1991.

Kapit, W., and L. M. Elson. (2001). *The Anatomy Coloring Book* (3rd ed.). San Francisco: Benjamin-Cummings Publishing Company, 2001.

Krasnow, D. Performance, movement, and kinesthesia. *Impulse, the International Journal of Dance Science, Medicine, and Education*, 2, 16–23, 1994.

Krasnow, D. H. C-I Training: The merger of conditioning and imagery as an alternative training methodology for dance. *Medical Problems of Performing Artists*, 12, 3–8, 1997.

Krasnow, D. H., and S. J. Chatfield. Dance science and the dance technique class. *Impulse, the International Journal of Dance Science, Medicine, and Education*, 4, 162-172, 1996.

Krasnow, D. H., S. J. Chatfield, S. Barr, J. L. Jensen, and J. S. Dufek. Imagery and conditioning practices for dancers. *Dance Research Journal*, 29/1, 43–64, 1997.

Krasnow, D., L. Mainwaring, and G. Kerr. Injury, stress, and perfectionism in young dancers and gymnasts. *Journal of Dance Medicine & Science*, 3, 51–58, 1999.

Krasnow, D. H., R. A. Monasterio, and S.J. Chatfield. Emerging concepts of posture and alignment. *Medical Problems of Performing Artists*, 16, 8–16, 2001.

Laws, K., and A. Sugano. *Physics and the Art of Dance: Understanding Movement* (2nd ed.). New York: Oxford Press, 2002.

Loman, S., and R. Brandt. (Eds.) *The Body-Mind Connection in Human Movement Analysis*. Keene, NH: Antioch New England Graduate School, 1992.

Matt, P. H. Ideokinesis: Integrating the science and somatics of dance. *Kinesiology and Medicine for Dance*, 14(1), 68–77, 1991–92.

Minton, S. Enhancement of alignment through imagery. *Journal of Physical Education, Recreation and Dance*, 61(2), 28–29, 1990.

Minton, S. Exploring the mind/body connection with imagery. *Kinesiology and Medicine for Dance*, 14(1), 29–32, 1991–92.

Netter, F. H. *Interactive Atlas of Human Anatomy* (CD-ROM). Summit, NJ: Ciba-Geigy, Medical Education and Publications, 1995.

Penrod, J. W., and J. G. Plastino. *The Dancer Prepares: Modern Dance for Beginners* (4th ed.). Mountain View, CA: Mayfield Publishing Company, 1998.

Pilates, J. H. *Return to Life through Contrology*. Boston: The Christopher Publishing House, 1945.

Rasch, P. *Kinesiology and Applied Anatomy*. Philadelphia: Lea & Febiger, 1989.

Rasch, P. J., and R. K. Burke. *Kinesiology and Applied Anatomy* (6th ed.). Philadelphia: Lea & Febiger, 1978.

Richardson, C., G. Jull, P. Hodges, and J. Hides. *Therapeutic Exercise for Spinal Segmental Stabilization in Low Back Pain: Scientific Basis and Clinical Approach*. Edinburgh: Churchill Livingstone, 1999.

Rommett, Z. *Personal Communication and Classroom Instruction from Ernest Pagano, Dancer and Teacher, in the Rommett Floor Barre Work*. New York: 1981–83.

Rommett, Z. *The Rommett Floor Barre Technique* [Video-recording]. New York: Zena Rommett Dance Association, 1991.

Ryan, A. J., and R. E. Stephens. *The Healthy Dancer: Dance Medicine for Dancers.* Princeton, NJ: Dance Horizon Books, 1987.

Ryman, R., and D. Ranney. A preliminary investigation of two variations of the grand battement devant. *Dance Research Journal*, 11, 2–11, 1979.

Shell, C. G. (Ed.). *The Dancer as Athlete*. Champaign, IL: Human Kinetics Publishers, Inc., 1986.

Shumway-Cook, A., and M. J. Wollacott. *Motor Control: Theory and Practical Applications* (2nd ed.). Baltimore, MD: Lippincott Williams & Williams, 2001.

Solomon, R. *Anatomy As a Master Image in Training Dancers* [Video-recording]. Santa Cruz, CA: Ruth Solomon, 1988.

Solomon, R., J. Solomon, and S. C. Minton. (Eds.). *Preventing Dance Injuries* (2nd ed.). Champaign, IL: Human Kinetics Books, 2005.

Spilken, T. *The Dancer's Foot Book*. Princeton, NJ: Princeton Book Company, 1990.

Sweigard, L. E. *Human Movement Potential: Its Ideokinetic Facilitation*. Lanham, MD: University Press of America, 1974.

Todd, M. E. *The Balancing of Forces in the Human Being: Its Application to Postural Patterns*. New York: Author, 1929.

Todd, M. E. *The Thinking Body: A Study of Balancing Forces of Dynamic Man*. New York: Paul B. Hoeber, Medical Book Department of Harper & Brothers, 1937.

Watkins, A., and P. M. Clarkson. *Dancing Longer, Dancing Stronger.* Princeton, NJ: Princeton Book Company, 1990.

Welsh, T. *Conditioning for Dancers.* Gainesville, FL: University Press of Florida, 2009.

Wilmerding, V., and D. Krasnow. Motor learning and teaching dance. Resource paper from the International Association for Dance Medicine & Science. Retrieved from <www.iadms.org/displaycommon.cfm?an=1&subarticlenbr=250>. 2009.

Index of Anatomical Terms

O

P

Q

R

S

T

U

V

W